*Dear Eva,
You are such a gift to this world.
Thank you for being you!
Love & Aloha,
Douglas*

MaKARA
A TASTE OF FREEDOM

DOUGLAS COONEY

Copyright © 2014 Douglas Cooney
PO Box 1918
Margaret River
WA   6285

Published by Vivid Publishing
P.O. Box 948, Fremantle
Western Australia 6959
www.vividpublishing.com.au

National Library of Australia Cataloguing-in-Publication data:
Author: Cooney, Douglas, author.
Title: Makara : a taste of freedom / Douglas Cooney.
ISBN: 9781925209082 (paperback)
Subjects: Surfers--Fiction.
          Surfing--Fiction.
Dewey Number: A823.4

Revised edition. All rights reserved. No part of this publication may be reproduced, stored in a retrieval system or transmitted in any form or by any means, electronic, mechanical, photocopying, recording or otherwise, without the prior written permission of the copyright holder.

This book is dedicated to anyone
who has the courage to share their unique
gifts with the world in any way, shape or form.
As a wise teacher once said,
"Don't die with your music still inside you."

1. GIRL'S BLOUSE

"Slow down Makara... slow down..." Citrine whispered, in her soft, goddess-like voice. "Take your time, this is not a race," she continued in a cute French accent, softly pressing him away.

The ferocious lion inside of him had come alive, ready to devour its prey. His heart beating so powerfully, it was almost exploding right out of his chest. Responding to her words, he retreated, but only a little, her musky scent hypnotically holding him close. He'd never been with such a gorgeous woman before. And here, on the grass, under the trees, with a cool, sparkling river flowing past, Makara was in paradise. The morning sun warmed his bare back and the way he was feeling right now, was something he'd only ever glimpsed before.

Slowly, easing his half naked body back down onto Citrine, he looked deeply into her sparkling, honey-coloured eyes. He was mesmerised. The finger tips of his right hand followed the folds of her shirt, gently stroking the side of her firm breast. Confidently he moved in to kiss her again. This time, she willingly received his lips. Electricity shot like rainbows of joy through their two young bodies, as they both surrendered to each other and to the energy of the moment. Citrine began moving sensually and breathing harder. Makara's blood was beginning to boil. His lion's paw reached down, intent on removing her top.

There was a short, loud knock on the door and Dave woke with a fright.

"Dave, wake up!" his mum yelled. "You'll be late for work!" He mumbled a few Neanderthal-sounding tones to acknowledge her and just lay there in amazement. *Where was I? Who was that beautiful woman? And why was she calling me Makara?* Energy poured through his body and his pulsating erection was that hard, it hurt. The experience seemed so real and he closed his eyes again, vividly recounting the scene.

Good old mum hey, he thought and then looked at his clock, realising it was already twenty to nine. A quick shower, a few muesli bars in the pocket, and he was out the door.

"Afternoon junior," Col said, in his usual dry pitch, finishing off a ciggy and spitting a dark coloured glob of un-healthiness at Dave's feet. Dave shook his head in disgust and dodged the landmine.

"Five minutes late and that's my greeting... Fuck you Col, ya old cunt."

"Watch ya lip there young fella or I'll knock ya block clean off, you hear," came the shaky reply.

"Yeah, you and whose army?" Col got up quickly and went to grab Dave, who was way too fast for him.

"You'll get yours young fella... you'll get yours," he shouted, chasing Dave for five metres before buckling over with his hands on his knees, out of breath and coughing, his face now bright red.

"Yeah, whatever," Dave said, not even bothering to look back and made for the stack of timber that still needed sorting from yesterday. He tripped on a piece of plastic. "Fuck this joint... and where does he get off treating me like that!"

The whole place was disorganised and under staffed. And with the Sydney Olympic preparations going on, the city had just gone into overdrive. Seemed everyone had the building bug. For a first job it paid kinda well though, but to be honest, it sucked. There definitely had to be more to life than mixing paint and stacking timber.

After an hour, Dave was exhausted. He headed for his favourite little hide out sanctuary in the back corner of the yard. It was concealed between the drying racks and had been well used lately. There was a big old gum tree hanging over the fence and a stack of four weathered pallets to sit on. He slumped down, head between his knees. A neat line of orange and black bull ants travelled passed the front of his boots, making for the fence. Dave just sat there, blankly observing their movements. They were so into what they were doing, his presence didn't seem to bother them at all.

"Ahh, caught ya slack arse, what da ya think ya doing just sittin' around?" blasted Col, red in the face again. "Just 'cause ya aunty works here, doesn't mean ya runnin' the show, ya hear me!" Col moved in closer, grabbing him by the scruff of the neck. Dave sprung up, forcefully breaking his grip.

"Don't you lay a finger on me old man... I'll fuck'n tear you apart!" Dave exploded, pushing the old alcoholic back into a stack of hardwood. Col rebounded, fists at the ready, shaping up for battle.

"C'mon ya little punk... What've you got... C'mon!"

Dave looked him straight in the eye and raised his open hands. The air was thick with rage.

"Back off Col! You don't wanna do this... You know what happened last time." Dave slowly walked backwards, trying his best to diffuse the situation and yet close to snapping himself.

"You're gutless. Look at ya. You young blokes these days. You've got nothin'!" he coughed, feeling somewhat victorious. It took Dave everything he had to surrender. In a way he felt sorry for the old bloke. Col spat one of his standard numbers onto the dirt, eased his guard and placed his weathered hands back on his hips. "If ya don't get that arse of yours back into gear shortly, I'll be havin' words with Ian, ya hear!"

Dave did his best to avoid Col for the rest of the day and finally it came to an end. With the most spark he'd had since arriving that morning, Dave bee-lined it for his little Mazda wagon on the far side of the car park. As he opened the door, he stopped for a moment to take in old Col limping back to the office. He'd been at the hardware store forty years and it seemed the daily monotony and the alcohol had just ruined him. He was an angry, empty shell of a man. Dave slowly sat down, inserting his keys into the ignition, eyes still fixed on the Aussie battler.

"Fuck this place!" Dave thundered, "There's no way I'm workin' here for the next forty years!"

The little wagon cranked over, throwing the usual cloud of white smoke into the air. He drove out of there, relieved another day was done. Weather wise, it had turned out to be an okay afternoon. The sun still had some summer warmth left in it but with the cool evenings, autumn was really starting to sink her teeth in.

I'll stop by the video store, Dave thought to himself, whilst sitting in the traffic at another red light. After all, he was looking down the barrel of another Saturday evening alone and needed some form of entertainment.

He pulled into the car park and was happy to see Bob's blue Kombi Van there. Bob worked in the video store and was an interesting, hippie kind of guy from California. A few of the local kids had nicknamed him Jesus 'cause of his long, matted brown hair and beard. Dave had been getting to know him over the last months and was always stoked to see him.

"Hey Bob, ya got any new movies that are kind of funny and light? I've had a wild day and I'm also sick of havin' nightmares," Dave said with a laugh.

"Sorry man, I'm afraid it's a sad state of affairs at the moment," Bob replied in his relaxed Californian drawl. "All the new ones are either killin' or relationship dramas of some description. You may want to check out the kid's section."

"You serious! Those days are long gone mate." Dave walked away from the counter, questioning Bob's sanity and thinking a comedy might just do the trick. His brother had recommended a good one but he couldn't quite remember the name. After a few minutes browsing, nothing jumped out at him.

Somehow, he ended up in kiddies corner and began flicking through the colourful array of options there. His pants began ringing loudly. Dave fumbled around, eventually answering:

"Hey Mikey, what are ya up to?"

"Nothin', just cruisin'. Did ya get a surf?"

"Nah... been on the work program. How was it?"

"Yeah, epic. Been surfin' all day. You comin' out tonight?"

"Nah, I'm knackered hey... reckon I'll have a quiety."

"Fuck mate, what's wrong with ya? You haven't been out for ages. You turnin' into the full girl's blouse or what?"

"Fuck off mate, you're the boogy boardin' blouse. No wonder ya can't even get a chick!" The phone went silent and Dave jumped back in: "Nah mate, I'm just over it... really. Been doin' the same thing every weekend since I was thirteen."

Again, silence haunted the phone. This time a little longer.

"Everyone's been wondering where ya are, that's all... It's different without ya, you know."

Dave felt a tightness in his throat. "Yeah, whatever Mikey. You're all so off ya heads, you wouldn't even know who's there anyway! I've got shit to do mate, so I'll see ya later."

"Righto, yeah, take care, see ya," Mikey said awkwardly, not expecting the call to finish so soon.

"See ya." Dave hung up, took a deep breath and stared vacantly at the shelves in front of him. *For fuck sake... It's Saturday arvo and here I am at the movie store, in the kids section! Have I totally lost it?*

Dave thought of his friends. He actually really missed them as well. He wondered what they'd be doing tonight. Well, he actually knew exactly what they'd be doing, 'cause he'd done it a hundred times before. All the lads would meet at Shane's house around five. From there the barby would be fired up and the beers would flow freely. Once everyone was sufficiently primed, they'd head for the local RSL club. This was a cross between a retirement village and a pub, but the beers were cheap, so it was a great place to hit before the next stage of the evening. From there, in a super drunken state, the night could unfold in various ways. Usually, everyone would end up in a mini-bus taxi heading to the nightclub, where all sorts of craziness would go down. Come Sunday morning about three or four was when your head would finally hit the pillow, unless of course you got lucky!

Far out, which movie to choose! What the fuck am I even doin' here? Dave questioned, snapping out of his daydream. He realised picking a movie wasn't going to happen and dawdled back to the counter, where Bob was sorting through some returns.

"Were you jokin' sendin' me to the kid's section, or what?" Dave asked, with some fire in his belly.

"Relax man... there are some hidden gems on those shelves. Things aren't always what they seem from the outside ya know. And guess what dude, I've found your movie. It comes with a no nightmare guarantee." Bob slowly lifted the video from behind the counter, building suspense with every movement. "*Tarzan!* It's a new one from Disney. Legendary tale, and they've even got some jungle surfin' goin' on in there. I just know you're gunna love it." He gently sat the movie down, realising his enthusiasm was falling on deaf ears. "You okay Dave? You're a bit out there today man?"

Dave squinted and shook his head a little.

"I just dunno what the fuck's happenin'... I feel like a walking ghost or somethin'. I hardly even had enough energy to work today and now I'm just rooted." Bob was all ears and allowed Dave to go on. "I heard the surf was pumpin' too and all my friends are over me 'cause I don't even go out with 'em any more." Dave reached out, picking up the movie and glanced briefly into Bob's concerned eyes.

"You've had yourself checked out haven't ya?"

"Yeah, I've almost been to every doctor in the city and no one knows what the fuck's goin' on."

"Keep your language down a bit man," Bob said quietly. "I don't what you scarin' off the customers."

"Sorry mate… It's just been goin' on for too long. It's doin' my head in. It sucks when even the doctors can't fix you up."

"Oh man, the medical system, that's a tricky one. Y'know the accident and emergency stuff is great… but these days, main stream doctors are only treatin' the symptoms and not the cause," Bob said in his peaceful manner. "If you get a big ol' crack in your garden hose and the water's sprayin' out, what's the very first step you take? Do you put some tape over the hole or do you go and turn the tap off?" He looked at Dave intently, awaiting an answer and soon realised he wasn't going to get one. He continued:

"Unfortunately, it's a sign of the times dude. Things are moving that fast, there is only time to whack a band aid on and get the next person through the door. Jeez… I'm glad I'm not a doctor. It's hectic enough in here come rush hour."

"Yeah, I'm hearin' ya mate… So what do I do then?"

"Man, probably stop worryin' about it all is the best place to start. They reckon stress is one of the biggest factors in health problems today. It kinda gets overlooked though, 'cause everyone's doin' it. It's almost seen as cool to be stressed, or productive or somethin'. It's just nuts. You know what I'm sayin'?"

"Yeah, old Col at work is the prime example of that. For sure, I hear ya."

Dave stepped to the side to let a father, daughter combo in to hire a few movies. Once they left, the shop was empty. Bob raised his voice a few more notches:

"So bro, I reckon you've just gotta learn to start listenin' to that body of yours some more. Make your health top priority. Rest when you're tired. Eat when you're hungry. Those simple things can take you a loooong way, ya know."

Dave was miles away again, lost in the bright colours of the video cover. Without even looking up, he mumbled to Bob:

"I'm knackered mate, I'm outta here," and began heading for the door. He jumped as Bob's voice of authority boomed out across the shop: "Not so fast man! I haven't even scanned that movie yet," he declared, bursting out with laughter. "I don't wanna have to call security on ya."

Dave returned to the counter with some more spring in his step. "Sorry mate," he said, handing the movie back and joined in with a little laugh. "Guess I am a bit out of it hey."

"There you go bro," Bob grinned, handing it back and throwing a play punch into his right shoulder.

"Aargh!" Dave yelped, "that hurt… " and moved back just enough to avoid any more blows.

"Sorry bro, sometimes I forget my own power… The reality is man, you've been through the wringer lately in more ways than one. You know, that whole scene with Anne, missin' out on Uni and this mystery sickness. Sometimes life just throws a bunch of stuff…" Dave's face turned the colour of recycled toilet paper and he leaned in, holding the counter with both hands, head spinning out of control, vision completely blurred. Bob raced around to help his friend but it was too late. Dave dropped to the ground like an old meat carcass onto the butcher shop floor. His legs wedged awkwardly against the wall.

"Dave. Dave. Can you hear me?" Bob said, shaking his shoulders. Nothing. Bob slid Dave away from the wall and lifted up his legs, jamming his arm under them to get some blood back to the brain. He shook him again, this time with more vigour. "Fuck Dave, wake up!" Still nothing. Bob stopped and took a deep breath to calm himself down. He'd done some first aid training years ago and remembered how important the airway was. There was a slight breath going on but he was in no position to check inside his mouth for any blockages. He began looking for the closest chair to use instead of his arm.

Out of the blue Dave returned. "How did I get down here?" he said, totally puzzled, rubbing his elbow.

"I'll just keep holdin' your legs up for a bit bro... Jesus! Thought I'd lost ya there man."

Dave lay there regrouping, while Bob kept questioning him just to make sure he remained present and wasn't going to pass out again. After five minutes Dave dragged himself up off the floor, with help from the big fella. Luckily no other customers came in during the drama. It would've looked a little strange.

"Last thing I heard you say was 'through the wringer', and then I started trippin' out. Fuck, that was gnarly." Bob grabbed a chair and slid it over.

"Here, sit down and take it easy for a bit bro. Do you want some water? I've got a banana here too."

"Yeah, that'd be good. Thanks."

Dave was very quiet, still in shock. He sat there sipping water and eating his banana. The store slowly began to fill with customers. Bob weaved his magic, all the while keeping an eye on his young friend. Eventually Dave felt ready to go. He needed a good feed and an early night. He'd hardly eaten all day. Just two muesli bars and a sandwich. Maybe that's why he'd passed out. Tomorrow was the start of his weekend, which he was thoroughly looking forward to. It had been a long day.

"I'm outta here mate. Thanks again for lookin' after me."

"Are you sure you'll be okay?"

"Yeah, I'm feelin' much better now. Not sure what all that was about. Reckon I just need to toughen up a bit."

Dave headed for the door. Bob beat him there and opened it for him.

"You take care man. Give this body of yours what it needs. I'd say a good rest is in order."

"Cheers, will do. See ya mate." Dave headed back to his car, shut the door and put his belt on. *Maybe I am turnin' into the full girl's blouse*, he pondered, shaking his head, upset with himself. It was one thing after another lately. Like he was caught in some endless spinning shit cycle. Dave pointed the Mazda for home.

It was weird. Bob had only been working at the movie store for the past six months but Dave felt as though he'd known him for years. The way they talked to each other was interesting and real... it was new. So refreshing to not be talking about the weather, footy, or who was drunkest from the night before – especially now, as he was off the party program. Bob was quite a bit older though, but it didn't seem to matter. They'd become good friends.

Dave pulled the fawn coloured wagon up outside his parents house. To the west, the sun was setting and the sky was alive with oranges and pinks and all sort of other crazy colours he didn't even have names for.

Since his health had taken a turn for the worse, he was finding more time to just stop and take things in. He had no choice really. His energy had just disappeared. There was no way a few months ago he would have been caught dead on a Saturday arvo just chilling in his car, watching the sunset, outside his folk's house. He was constantly struggling with the idea, that this is not the way a nineteen year old ought to live.

Dave's Mum, Dad and sister had all gone out for the evening and would not be home till around ten or eleven. His brother Sean would be well under way with the post football celebrations, which meant that tonight Dave had the house to himself. This freaked him out a bit 'cause if he passed out again there was no one around to help.

So there he was, sitting alone in the car outside his parent's house, as the last colours of the sunset began to fade. Already a couple of stars had begun to poke out their heads. Night was on its way.

Dave drifted off into thoughts of Anne, his girlfriend... well, now ex-girlfriend. A wave of anger passed through him, slowly rippling out into a deep loneliness. His heart felt heavy and there was a pain in his throat.

"Fuck her! Why did she leave me? What did I do wrong?" he roared into the silence, directing a stern blow into the steering wheel with both palms. A couple of tears slid down his face, landing silently on the dusty, blue uniform. His whole world was falling apart. The last time he'd cried was when he broke his wrist playing rugby in Year 9 at school and that was because the pain was so intense. He'd managed to keep it together pretty well since Anne had dumped him. Just been doing his best to not even think about her.

Suddenly a car pulled into next door's driveway, not too far from where he was parked. Dave quickly wiped away his tears and pulled himself together. He waited for them to go in first and when it was safe, jumped out of the car and made for the front door. It was almost dark now.

He hadn't eaten anything solid since lunch and was ravenous. He opened the freezer to dig out a frozen pie. A few minutes in the microwave while he had a shower and dinner would be on. In his recent quest for better health, he was beginning to understand the classic, 'you are what you eat' saying. But old habits die hard and the faithful frozen pie had been a good friend for years.

Perhaps some of last night's salad with it could help even the score, he thought, as he heard the microwave beeping its ready signal from the shower.

The pie and salad were demolished in a few minutes. Dave strolled into the lounge room to get comfy in his favourite couch and put the video on. Dinner had done wonders and he felt much better. It actually turned out to be quite a good movie, containing some uplifting messages which surprised him. He'd not expected that from a kid's show... especially *Tarzan*. It was exactly what he was needing and for a while forgot all about his misery.

"Good call Bob!" he said out loud, instantly feeling a bit odd for talking with no one around.

It had been a long, intense day and he was exhausted. The time was 9 p.m. and he was ready to hit the hay. His elbow throbbed from where he'd fallen on it and there was some pain in his wrist as well. It was minimal damage compared to the last time he'd passed out, so he wasn't too concerned.

Dave felt his head heavy on the pillow and smiled, eyes darting around the room at the magnificent collage of surfing posters all over his walls.

"What would it take for me to get back in the water?" he questioned out loud again, enjoying it this time. "I'm sooooo ready for a change."

The quiet of the house was relaxing and a little unusual at the same time. Dave reached over and turned out the light. His body sank into the soft, warm bed and within seconds he was off to sleep.

2. LETTING GO

Dave awoke startled, to a soft tapping noise on his window. Still dark outside. It couldn't be a bird, they weren't even up yet. Next came a short, sharp whisper:

"Dave, Dave... you in there?"

In a split second he froze, breathing stopped, his body still and quiet as possible. Transported to five years old again, terrified of the darkness and the impending attack from the monster under his bed. Silently, squeezing a few shallow breaths, the initial adrenalin boost subsided and his rational mind kicked in. *Whoever this is knows my name*, he reasoned and the fear instantly melted away.

The voice came again and this time it sounded familiar:

"Dave, wake up, it's me."

"Yeah, yeah... give me a sec," Dave replied quietly, as he sat up and took a fuller breath. He opened the curtains. It was Bob.

"What the hell are you doin' here? It's pitch fuckin' black!" Dave said surprised, trying not to raise his voice too much.

"Sorry to startle you man, but it's all part of the grand plan."

"What grand plan? What's the time? You been drinkin'?"

"I'm straight as man. I don't even drink. We're goin' on an adventure. We could be gone for a few weeks. Grab some warm clothes, your favourite surfboard and don't forget your wetsuit. I'll meet you out the front at my van. We leave in five minutes!" finished Bob, with a tone of authority and sharpness in his voice that was very unlike him.

"Bob... Bob..." Dave whispered, with his nose jammed against the fly-screen. It was too late. The long haired, yankee madman had already disappeared into the darkness.

This is fucked up! he thought, switching the light on, trying to grasp what the hell was happening. Yes it was fucked up... but a sudden aliveness was dancing in his belly. He randomly began jamming clothes into his bag, trying to be as quiet as a mouse. A hundred questions flicked through his head. *Where are we goin'? What about work? Am I losing my mind doin' this?*

Rubbing the sleep from his eyes, he looked down at his backpack which lay on the floor in front of him.

It was loaded and ready to go. Dave opened the desk drawer and grabbed his savings from underneath a stack of surf mags. The recent total was $420. He took it all and tucked it into the front zipper compartment of his pack.

Five minutes was getting close and he didn't want to keep Bob waiting. He turned off the light and silently tip-toed down the hallway. As he passed through the kitchen, he wrote a small note to his parents on the back of an envelope that was sitting on the bench.

Hey Mum and Dad, I've gone on a surf trip with Bob from the movie store. I'll see you a bit later. Dave

He walked across the wet lawn to the garden shed and after rustling around in the dark, finally found his surfboard and wetsuit, both of which hadn't been used in a long time. As he awkwardly backed out through the door it closed with an unexpected bang, the sound echoing out through the neighbourhood. *Fuck! The old man will be out here with his stick if I keep this up.* He decided to move a little quicker just in case. The air was fresh and icy and the stars were still shining. To the east, a feint orange glow signalled the arrival of a new day.

Dave was ready. Backpack on. Board and wetsuit under his arm. As he jogged passed the clothesline, he dragged off his brother's cold, wet beach towel. Dave hadn't been up before the sunrise for months. It was so quiet. A real serenity in the air. As he arrived at the front of the house, he was greeted by Bob and his classic van.

"Put your board in here dude," he said, sliding open the side door.

Dave didn't respond... he just stood there, suddenly frozen... not knowing what to do. This was all so unplanned... his mind was going bananas. He had questions, doubts, fears and so much more all coming to the surface at once.

How did Bob even know where I live? What am I getting myself into here? Bob's two large hands firmly grabbed Dave by the shoulders and gave him a shake.

"Snap out of it man! It's freezing out here. Throw your stuff in and let's get on the road. You need this!" exclaimed Bob, with that same authority in his voice as before. A big smile came to Dave's face and again he felt a light wave of excitement pass through his body.

"Yes, I do need this," he said quietly, but with strength in his voice.

With that, he lay his board down in the back of the Kombi and carefully placed his pack next to a box filled with books. He'd never seen inside Bob's van before and even in the dark he could make out where the kitchen was, complete with a cute little fridge. The cupboards were covered with a variety of photos and artworks. And the smell... the smell was like a natural perfume. The same smell you get in those hippie shops. It was strong, but quite nice. For such a small space there was definitely a lot going on. To

Dave's surprise it was all neat and very well organised. It felt like a colourful little home on wheels.

The engine rattled to life and Dave slid the side door shut with a thud. He then climbed up into the passenger's seat and they were away. He still had a hundred and ten questions on the tip of his tongue, but knew that right now wasn't the time to ask. The stereo pumped with some funky, relaxing beats that Dave recognised from an old surf movie he'd watched a few times. It was a comfy van to travel in. Much noisier than his Mazda wagon but it felt solid and spacious and the windscreen was huge, so you were able to get a good view of the road ahead.

They were heading south and the city streets were quiet, which was refreshing for a change. Bob hadn't said a word since they'd left the house and Dave was starting to become uncomfortable. He reached down to check his phone and then realised he'd left it at home in the rush to leave.

"Bob, I've left my phone behind!"

"Just forget about it man. It's probably a blessing in disguise. I've got my doubts about those things anyway," he replied, sounding a bit more like his usual calm self, "Sorry Dave, I was a bit sharp with you back at the house man, but I felt it was necessary to get you movin'."

"Yeah, that's cool. It worked. But to be honest, I don't even know where we're goin'. You haven't told me fuck all." Dave said, looking sternly across at Bob.

"Fair enough… I reckon I'd be pissed too if someone came tappin' on my window at 5 a.m. It was out of left field dude and I'm sorry but that's the way I roll. I just love doin' crazy shit!" Bob laughed, doing his best to lighten things up. Dave relaxed a little, but still had his questions:

"So, where are we goin'? And for how long? I'm workin' Tuesday and didn't even get a chance to speak with me oldies about this."

"Relax, it's all been taken care of bro. You've been comin' into the store for the past few months with a broken heart, health concerns, low energy and a bunch of other stuff. So I've taken it upon myself to help you out. Your folks know exactly what's happenin' and your Mum's arranged with your Aunt for you to take a vacation.

"When I was your age my life wasn't goin' too good either, and a friend took me on a surfin' adventure away from the city. It changed my life forever... We're headin' down to my brother's place, 'bout three hours from here. He has an awesome 'eco house' in the bush and nearby there are some great waves. You'll love it dude! A change of scenery and some fresh air is the best medicine for you right now, so just kick on back and enjoy the ride."

Dave sat there, stunned with Bob's words. Everything had been organised and he was none the wiser. Normally he was on the pulse at sniffing out surprises but this one had definitely snuck up on him. He felt like he was on the verge of laughing and crying and then just started feeling plain old weird. Why was Bob doing this for him? What had he done to deserve this?

"Wow, you're a legend Bob. We ain't even known each other that long and you've done all this for me. To be honest, I'm really blown away. Thanks mate." It was almost too much to receive. He knew Bob was a good guy but this little stunt had truly taken the cake. A big smile of gratitude came to his face and his body was instanly warm.

"No worries mate!" Bob replied, throwing in a dodgy Aussie accent. Dave's body relaxed some more and excitement started to move through him again. He was feeling different but couldn't quite put his finger on what it was.

They'd gone through the Harbour tunnel and the main part of the city. The traffic was starting to thicken up and they were now on the highway heading through the southern suburbs. The houses were all stacked closely together. Barely a tree in sight. The sun was just starting to show it's golden rays through the dense morning fog.

The dashboard of the van was filled with random shells and colourful stones. There was even this cute, little green Buddha statue, with springs on its legs and every time they hit a bump, it would groove into a selection of wild dance moves. The stereo continued to pump and Dave was enjoying the music a lot. Sometimes it actually looked like the Buddha was dancing to the rhythm of the song.

Bob reached back into a bag behind his seat and pulled out some fruit.

"Want an apple?"

"Yeah, thanks mate. I was gettin' a bit hungry."

Dave took a bite and there was an explosion of taste in his mouth. It was crisp, juicy and his tongue was left buzzing.

"Wow! Where did these babies come from?" he enquired with enthusiasm.

"You know that funky little organic fruit and veg shop, just down from the movie store. They had a fresh delivery yesterday and oohh man, I just couldn't resist... I love a good apple and by the sounds of it you do too."

"Yeah... Best ever apple without a doubt," Dave said, taking a second bite which was even better than the first. "I've never even been into that shop, might be worth a look."

His Mum and Dad had gone there to check it out when it first opened but were totally shocked with the prices and never went back. That's why Dave hadn't even been in there. Seemed like it was just a rip-off shop, taking advantage of people. He didn't even know what organic meant.

The houses had now given way to the majestic National Park and the city was becoming a distant vision behind them. Dave turned and looked through the rear window of the van. He could see the shapes of the larger city buildings, a brown haze surrounding them. They almost looked blood orange in the morning light. As Dave turned back towards the front, he breathed in an ocean of green trees and a weight lifted from his shoulders.

Bob sensed a shift and without much thought

wound down his window, letting in the freezing morning air and screamed with all his lung power: "Yooooouuuuuhooooooooooo!!!" until he was completely out of breath and quickly wound the window back up, laughing uncontrollably.

"I've been kidnapped by a nut case," Dave responded, with a smile and a few half chuckles, attempting to join in on the fun. Bob had this wild, full belly laugh, that was out of control. It was loud and non stop. A bit intimidating for Dave, who wondered what all the fuss was about. Bob laughed and laughed – It was a crazy scene, flying down the highway in the old blue Kombi, with an acid fuelled Jesus at the wheel.

"This could be a good time to introduce you to my old friend and travellin' buddy, 'Freedom'," Bob announced, bursting with energy, acting like he was making an official speech. "Dave... this is Freedom," he said, rubbing his hand lovingly over the dashboard in front of the steering wheel. "And Freedom... meet Dave," Bob said, with a hand gesture towards Dave and two short bursts of the horn. "I was going to introduce you two earlier... but in the right moment things happen and this definitely feels like the right moment."

"Very pleased to meet you Freedom," Dave replied, starting to enjoy the weirdness and play along. "I have a feelin' we're goin'-to-get-on like a house on fire."

They'd barely been gone an hour and already Dave was beginning to feel better than he had in a long time.

LETTING GO

Since his last year at High school and then working full-time, he'd been so busy that he hadn't even left the city once. In his younger years, the family was always going on holidays and adventures which he really loved, but for one reason or another, they'd just slipped out of the picture.

The day was in full swing now, with the morning sun lighting up a clear, blue sky. The fog and low cloud had melted away, revealing a classic autumn day.

"How does it get any better than this?" Bob exclaimed excitedly. "I was just cuttin' ties with the city and my work. It's a really cool little exercise to do when you're startin' a new adventure. Want me to run you through it?"

"Maybe... what's it all about?" Dave asked defensively.

"So you generally close your eyes... a little hard for me right now," he laughed, "Then you visualise in front of you, whatever you feel could be holdin' some of your energy or thoughts. For instance, a couple of good ones for you would be the hardware store, or your ex-girlfriend."

"Dunno mate, it all sounds a bit fuckin' strange to me... ya reckon it could help?"

"I've no doubt dude. Ya might just have to trust me on this one."

"Righto... I'll give it a crack then," Dave said, rubbing his hands together in preparation.

"Great man... and you can relax, you're not gunna end up like me, don't worry. So... once you've got what you want to let go of in front of you, the next step is to feel or visualise any cords, connections, chains, or anythin' else that is tyin' you to whatever's there. Make it like a fun game and use your imagination... it really works. Anyway, let's give it a shot. Who would you like to do first?"

"Let's start with the hardware," Dave said, excitement in his voice.

"Okay, so close your eyes and visualise the hardware store in front of you... got it?"

"Yep, got it."

"Okay, so next see or feel whatever's holdin' you to it. Can you get a sense of what's there?"

"It's wild! I can picture the store really clearly and there are dozens of white ropes comin' from the posts on the front verandah, and they're connected to my legs, arms, everywhere."

"Awesome, you've got a good imagination. Next step is cutting the ropes. You can use whatever comes to you. Scissors, a knife, an axe... sometimes I even get a picture of a samurai warrior cuttin' the cords. There's no limit on how creative you can be. The main thing is just to cut those suckers!"

"Oh my God!" Dave laughed. "It's old Col and he's goin' at the ropes with a chainsaw. He's actually goin' bananas. I've never seen him move like that before." Dave continued, laughing until all the ropes were cut. "This is out of control Bob. The whole store is liftin' off the ground and floatin' up into the sky, and shrinkin' at the same time. Far out, a pair of massive wings have grown out from each side and it's flyin' away!"

LETTING GO

Dave's laughter fell silent as he slowly watched the hardware store flying off into the distance, until it completely disappeared. As soon as it vanished, a feeling of lightness passed through him and a huge relief that he wasn't expecting.

"Mate. Are you sure those apples we ate earlier were just normal apples? That was just out there, but at the same time somethin' really happened. I feel different."

"Yeah, I really like that one," Bob said, happy Dave have given it a go. "It's just so easy. It seems we leave bits and pieces of ourselves energetically here, there and everywhere and it's a great practice to do, to become more whole, present and energised. Man, wait till you try it with your ex-girlfriend... and as for those apples, they definitely weren't normal. They were missin' a coating of wax and pesticide spray," he laughed again.

Dave didn't even hear what Bob had said. As soon as he mentioned doing it with his ex-girlfriend he'd closed his eyes and began the process again.

Oh, Anne... For the past two years they'd been together and had an awesome time. This was Dave's first long-term relationship and he'd come to the conclusion that Anne was the one. They shared so much in common and he still couldn't imagine life without her. She'd taken off to Europe four months ago for a student exchange program in Germany, which altogether would last one year. The plan was for Dave to save up some dollars and head over there to meet her after six months.

One month after Anne had left, she emailed Dave and broke off the relationship. She'd fallen in love with some English guy at the language school and that was that! Dave was shell shocked. This totally broke his heart like it had never been broken before. He just couldn't believe it'd happened to him. Even now, after three months, he could still feel a pain in his chest. He wanted to jump on a plane to go and see her and try to sort things out. And to find this Pommy pansy, the Queens nephew, or whoever he was, and rip his head off. Unfortunately he hadn't managed to save enough money and with this mystery illness haunting him, there was no way it was going to happen. This cut him deeply. He longed to be the knight in shining armour, that would sail across the seas to reclaim his true love.

Dave focused hard and visualised her sitting in front of him. So beautiful... For the next five minutes he remained silent, deeply in his own world, cutting ties with Anne and freeing the burden that had been weighing him down so heavily. Bob knew what he was up to and remained quiet at the wheel, carrying on down the highway.

Tears began to flow down Dave's cheeks in a constant trickle. The pain in his heart had returned and he was deep in the process of letting go. He'd been amazed at the amount of ties there were, and to all parts of his body. He'd been gently going through and cutting each one with a pair of golden scissors.

One cord to his heart remained and he was struggling to cut it. How could he let her go? She had meant so much to him and there still could be... SNIP! The last cord fell to the ground in front of him and as he looked up, Anne was no longer there. Where had she gone? Had he killed her? Was she okay?

"She's gone Bob... she's just vanished," he said softly, wiping the tears from his face, feeling a bit self-conscious.

"Yeah man... sometimes we just gotta let 'em go."

"It's weird though, 'cause I still love her," Dave said, sniffling and shaking his head.

"That's okay... you'll never stop lovin' her man, but it's no use hangin' on. You've gotta free yourself up for the next goddess."

Dave went silent again and closed his eyes, attempting to grasp what had just happened... Eventually the questions vanished and the tears stopped flowing. He'd done it! A raw and vulnerable shakiness consumed his entire body. At the same time, a small candle flame of joy which had been gone for months, started burning once again. Only a little flame, but it was enough to bring some hope to his watery eyes.

"This hippie shit is powerful," Dave laughed.

"Man... you ain't seen nothin' yet!"

3. OUT THERE

It was a good time to pull over and Bob guided Freedom into a rest stop on the side of the highway. The dense, green forest they were travelling through was breathtaking. It would be a relief to get out and stretch the legs. He often stopped here on his trips to the South Coast.

"You alright now Dave?"

"Yeah, thanks mate. It's been an intense mornin' hey, and I think that last exercise just topped it off. I've never cried so much in all my life. Don't know what's happenin' to me."

"You know man, a friend once told me that tears are the heart speakin' and I fully believe that's true. So it's awesome that you just let 'em come. They're precious gifts ya know. It also takes a lot of courage, because blokes don't cry right… especially Aussie blokes!" Bob said, finishing in his dodgy Australian accent, laughing.

"Yeah, guess you're right. Not so sure 'bout the heart speakin' bit though. It's just strange, like I've got no control over the tears comin'. I just feel like a skirt wearer or somethin'."

"It's not worth beatin' yourself all up about it man. And wearin' a skirt ain't the end of the world either, ya know! No stress dude. Your secret's safe with me. Just lighten' up a little. The amount of tears that have come out of these eyes over the years… far out, talk about fillin' a swimmin' pool."

"What've you had to cry about? You seem like you've got your shit together."

Bob looked across at Dave with big eyes, shaking his head: "Man… don't even get me started. Let's just say, we've got a lot more in common than you even realise. This is stage one of the healin' journey bro. You know this facade, this armour of toughness all us guys carry around. It's all bullshit, it's all ego. And the sooner that falls away, the sooner we can really start to live. As the tough shell crumbles, the tears flow on out… Years and years of holding back the rain, and eventually that damn gotta burst man. It's actually a real blessing that it's happenin' for ya. Some guys carry that shit to the grave."

"So it's a good thing," Dave questioned, now quite confused.

"Of course it is… I know it don't seem like it right now, but those tears are the start of your liberation man. Who wants to go through life carryin' around bucket loads of sad water anyway... And this whole being tough trip. The sooner you let that go, the better. All that shit weighs a tonne man.

"It's natural for us men to not feel though... We're the ones that have to go to war. We're the ones that have to be ready to kill. In a way, through the generations we've trained ourselves not to feel. But these days are different. You know what real strength is dude? Real strength is havin' the courage to drop that armour and face those feelings head on. To say, hey, I'm not runnin' from you, or shuttin' you out any more... like what you just did with Anne. That takes real guts bro. That's a true warrior." Dave nodded his head, humbly receiving the praise.

"So you're sayin', bein' tough isn't really bein' tough at all."

"Well, we think it is. But when it falls away you soon realise the illusion. And this armour doesn't just keep the tears away either... It stops us from feelin' in general. I mean everything; Happiness, anger, love, jealousy, ease... the list goes on dude. The deal is, if ya can drop that hard shell, life really opens up for you. Your experience of the world becomes richer and more alive than you ever imagined."

Bob opened his door and jumped out. It was a beautiful day. Dave sat there, trying to grasp what had just been revealed. It was true. For as long as he could remember, he'd done his best not to cry, especially not in front of anyone. That was a guaranteed death sentence. And imagine not having to be tough… that's real strength. His mind wrestled with the concept. Dave sighted Bob taking a piss and that's exactly what he was needing.

Was great to be outside and even better to have an empty. Towering gum trees surrounded them and the air was fresh and alive. You could even smell the eucalyptus. Dave took a few good deep breaths and relaxed into the day. His overloaded mind starting to unravel itself. The morning sun warmed his face and he actually felt pretty good. In the car park, Bob was performing a bunch of random body movements that were quite entertaining. There were a few rugby style warm ups, combined with stretches, some dance moves and some wild, full body shaking. It was very amusing for the young travelling companion to witness.

Next on the agenda was breakfast, which Bob took seriously. He busted out a container of his home made muesli, bowls, spoons, almond milk and a variety of other small paper bags, which held an assortment of special nuts and dried berries. It was quite a ceremony and he even layed out a rug in the sunshine, complete with a cushion each to sit on. Nothing was overlooked.

It was well worth it. The muesli was delicious. Dave wondered to himself how on earth they got milk from almonds. He was pretty certain that milk only came from cows and wanted to ask Bob but thought it was a stupid question. And he'd never even seen or heard of half the things in the muesli mix, but either way, it was tasty.

Another hour down the road, after some interesting discussions and more laughter, they arrived at a small town. Apparently Bob's brother lived only 25 minutes away. Freedom was needing some fuel and Bob pulled up at the first service station they saw. While he refuelled, Dave had an urge to help out and wiped the windscreen clean. It was needing some attention after collecting bugs all morning and Bob was grateful for the contribution.

Dave became uneasy. He wanted to pitch in for the fuel costs and at the same time realised he only had $420 to his name. His mind raced again with questions: How long would they be away for? Did they need to pay rent at Bob's brother's place? Did he need to save all his money for petrol costs?

"Bob, I'm really concerned about the money situation. I've only got $400 and I'm not sure how long it's gunna last."

"Relax bro... for now it's all taken care of. Your folks gave me $100 to help with fuel costs and your Aunt also pitched in $50. I figured we'd go halves in the fuel so I've got this old sock here as the kitty. Your $150 is in there and I've put $150 in too. So altogether, we have hundreds of kilometres up our sleeves. And as far as my brother's place goes: he's loaded! It won't cost us a dime... I mean, a cent."

"Fuckin' hell, you've done it again Bob," Dave said, fully baffled. "I really can't understand why you're doin' all this for me. It's amazing. I don't even know what to say."

"Like I said, someone did this for me once before

and I feel it's time to return the favour. On this adventure man, money will not be an issue. We are two creative, limitless beings, and if we can both really begin to trust life, we will be supported every step of the way. That's a guarantee."

Dave smiled at Bob and walked over to drop the beat up squeegee back into the yellow bucket. He hadn't heard anyone speak like this before. He was shocked, confused and doubtful all at the same time. *Could this really be possible? Money not being a problem.* It had been one surprise after the other today. Dave had barely even had a chance to think about being sick or his energy levels. He'd also left all of his medicine at home in the rush to leave. Far out… even his phone as well.

Dave jumped back in the Kombi while Bob went and sorted out the bill. As he glanced up to take in the action unfolding in this cute little town, he was surprised by three gorgeous girls walking by. They were literally only two metres away, and were really interested in the old blue Kombi, and possibly the guy in the passenger seat. Three glowing, big smiles hit him like a road train. The blonde girl in the red top, even turned and waved after they'd passed by. Dave just smiled nervously and waved back, at which all three of them giggled. Something like that hadn't happened for a long time and it left him feeling all tingly inside.

I might have to look at getting one of these vans, he thought to himself with a smile. *The little Mazda never gets that sort of reaction.*

Dave relayed the story with enthusiasm to his wild looking friend, who was stoked to hear it. Bob explained the whereabouts of an epic beach between the township and his brother's place. With the conditions as they were, there was a very good chance the surf would be pumping. The sun was shining. A light, autumn, off-shore breeze was rustling through the tree tops and a sense of excitement oozed through the van.

Freedom pulled into the dirt car park behind the sand dunes. Would Dave surf today? He'd been out of the water for a couple of months. Was he ready? Maybe a walk on the beach would be enough? Again, so many questions.

Dave had learned to surf when he was six years old with his Dad, who'd found an old surfboard on one of his building jobs that the owner had gladly given up. He'd taken Dave to a beginner's surf beach, about half an hour from where they lived. It was a perfect, warm summer's afternoon, with a knee-high, rolling wave in the southern corner. The very first whitewater that Dave's dad helped him into, he stood up straight away and rode it all the way to shore. The rest of the family were on the beach cheering and the smile on his young melon was so big, you could've seen it from the Harbour bridge.

From that moment on, Dave's life had revolved around the ocean and surfing. He just loved spending time at the beach. Riding waves was all he wanted to do. The freedom, the self-expression, the sun, the salt water and the challenging environment gave him so much joy.

In anticipation of what was to come, both Bob and Dave sprung out of the van and began jogging up the bush track through the dunes. They surprised a huge goanna walking across the path, which took off like a bullet once it saw them. As they got to the top of the hill, they were greeted by a sparkling, blue-green ocean, producing some fun little waves, fanned by a light wind. There was only a handful of other surfers scattered across the whole beach.

Dave took a deep breath in. The late morning sun had taken the icy chill out of the air. It was a beautiful scene that lay before him. He'd come to this area when he was younger but this particular beach was new to him.

"Wow! What a place," he said to Bob and breathed out, relaxing, feeling his bare feet on the cool sand. He hadn't felt sand beneath his feet for a while, that was for sure. "I feel so free, it's been way too long." Dave flashed on the last few months, and wondered where he'd been. He turned and looked Bob straight in the eyes. "I'm ready Bob, let's get out there."

"Fantastic bro. The comeback is on! Yeeewwwwww!" Bob howled, as he turned to run back down the track towards the van.

In no time, wetties were pulled on, boards waxed and they were running back up over the sand dunes, primed for action. Dave felt an invigorating new spring in his step. He was laughing and singing as he ran towards the ocean. Yes... something was definitely happening. Bob ran beside him, taking the whole scene in with amazement. He knew exactly what Dave was capable of and he also knew that this was just the beginning.

Dave didn't even bother to do his pre-surf stretch routine, he was far too excited for that. His youthful enthusiasm was back and he was truly celebrating it. The leg rope went on quickly and without even thinking, he was already lying on his board stroking through the glistening water, eyes on a perfect little beach break peak, that no one was surfing.

The water felt soooo good! It was super refreshing but not too cold and Dave's wetsuit kept him toasty. He was back on the horse. Feeling alive and energised. Within minutes, he was out the back and could see a great wave coming that had his name written all over it. His years of experience helped him to be exactly in the right spot at the right time. Next thing he knew, he was up and riding across a clean, shoulder-high right hander, with a smile from ear to ear.

"Yahhooooooooo!" he screamed as the wave finished, his smile now even bigger than before. He sat down on his board in the water and turned to look at Bob, who was stretching it up on the beach and screamed again, "Whoooooooweeee!" Bob returned with an equally crazy scream: "Yooyooyooyoo...yoooooooo!" and burst out laughing, throwing his fists up into the air, and breaking into a little dance, all in celebration of Dave's surfing comeback.

It wasn't long before Bob joined Dave in the lineup. He paddled over to his buzzing young friend and threw a massive high five at him. "Right on man! That's what I'm talkin' about!" Bob expressed, with all his heart. "You're rippin' these waves apart dude. Your gunna put this old bloke to shame."

"No chance old mate... Fuck... so good to be back in the water," Dave said, running his hands up over his face and through his hair. A good looking wave popped up and the lads scrambled for position. "Lets split this one hey Bob."

"Righto man, I'll go left." The wave picked them both up at the same time and they took off. Dave went right and Bob took the left. It was a clean, head-high wave that rattled off perfectly in either direction. With all the hooting and screaming, the other surfers down the beach probably wondered what the hell was going on.

Over the next hour, they split a bunch more peaks and surfed their brains out. Sharing stories in-between waves and even rode a few side by side, laughing the whole way. It was an all-time session and they had a blast.

Back at the van, Dave was exhausted and had a strong headache going on. Bob questioned him about his water intake and organised some immediately.

"Sometimes we forget about the simple things," he said to Dave, passing him some water.

"Yeah true, thanks Bob," he said, taking a huge drink from the bottle. "Wow! That's really good. I was needing that, thanks."

"No worries mate!" played Bob, putting on his not-so-good Aussie accent yet again and then returned to his normal voice. "I've got this hi-tech filter at home which takes out all the crap and then puts minerals back in. It even energises the water. Makes a difference don't ya reckon?"

"Definitely. And it's nice in a glass bottle for a change," Dave replied.

"Man, don't even get me started on that whole plastic thing! I was up in Indonesia last year and it was outta control. One place we were surfin' the water was just thick with the stuff. Some scientists even reckon the chemicals being released are changin' the sex of fish and stuff. Can you believe it? Imagine what it's doin' to us humans!" Bob said in disbelief.

"Changin' the sex of fish. Are you serious?"

"You bet man. I ain't got the full scoop on it... but it's food for thought."

The lads were starving after their surf session and Bob got in, popped the roof of the Kombi up and began to prepare lunch. Out of his little fridge came a plethora of things. Lettuce, sprouts, a carrot, beetroot, avocado and the list just went on. It was all so colourful and alive. Bob dived straight into creation mode and enlisted his partners help. Dave grated the carrot and fresh beetroot, ending up with a very purple hand. He'd only ever had beetroot in a can before and never overly enjoyed it. This stuff looked really juicy and his body was saying YES!

The final lunch creation was out of this world. Bob included a variety of nuts and seeds and even some salt he reckoned came from the Himalayan Mountains, that was supposed to be good for you. Dave had trouble believing that one. It was a taste sensation though and both the plates were emptied in no time at all.

Even though Dave was still knackered, his headache had eased a lot and he was starting to feel much better. Bob was really looking forward to seeing his brother and the family, so after a quick clean-up they were on the road again. Dave nodded off straight away in the passenger's seat.

4. FOR REST

Bob slowed down to pull into his brother's driveway. The van hit a big pot-hole and Dave's head bashed into the window he was sleeping against. He woke with a shock and half wondered where on earth he was... looking up with blurred eyes to get his bearings, he saw a big wooden sign, which read: FOR REST ECO RETREAT. *This must be it*, he thought, rubbing his head and eyes, and straightening himself up to get comfortable.

"Jeeez, you alright dude. That was one hell of a knock." Dave's vision was now completely back and he glanced over at the driver.

"Yeah mate. Tough as nails, remember," he said, with a cheeky smile.

"Sorry man, almost forgot." Freedom came to a

stop right in front of the sign. "Pretty cool, huh Dave. Sam came up with that sitting alone in the forest one day and saw the ancient message in the words. The forest... for-rest.... a place we go for rest, do you get it?"

"Mate, the knock on the head wasn't that bad. Of course I fuckin' get it! You don't have to spell it out like I'm in kindergarten."

"Take a breath, simmer down man... I'm just doin' the polite tour guide thing. I appreciate your feedback but you don't have to get all agro on me." Bob took a deep breath in and let a wild, grunting noise out. It sounded like a dirt bike starting up.

"You're one strange character that's for sure," Dave said, still angry and a bit disturbed by Bob's outburst.

"You're not wrong there my man. And I'm all good with strange... Okay, on with the tour. So what I was sayin' was, there are some great bush walks around this property. It's huge! The healin' power of these trees is phenomenal and I recommend you soak 'em up while your here dude. If they've got no bookings at the moment we'll have our own style'n cabin each, which'd be awesome. You look like you need a good rest. I reckon this is just what the doctor ordered."

"Yeah... it's true," Dave said, softening a little. "Sorry for bitin' your head off mate."

"All good man. Apology accepted and no offence taken."

Dave smiled and up the driveway they went. It was a dirt track surrounded by thick bush, which eventually opened up into a beautiful big clearing, revealing an earthy two-storey cottage up on a hill, surrounded by healthy looking trees and gardens. There were a couple of cute cabins off to the left. Dave guessed they were the ones Bob had just mentioned. It was a magical looking place and Dave instantly felt at home.

Bob pulled Freedom up behind a flashy-looking four wheel drive and two kids came racing out from behind the house. They were screaming Bob's name, laughing and coming straight for the van at top speed. Bob quickly exited and they both jumped up onto him, giving him a cross between some complex wrestling move and a hug. They were so excited to see their uncle and he was equally happy to see them. When the energy died down a little, Bob gave the official introduction.

"Sandy, Jarrah, this is my good friend Dave. Dave, this…" The kids let go of Bob and launched straight at Dave with the same manoeuvre. Bob was in stitches laughing and Dave, who wasn't expecting it, almost fell flat on his ass but somehow managed to keep his feet.

Sandy was probably about six and the little boy Jarrah, around three or four. They were clutching onto Dave and along with Bob, they laughed and laughed. Dave wasn't so sure about it all. They both looked him in the eye, to really check him out. He was mesmerised by their alive glow and the shine in their eyes. He'd definitely never seen kids like this before. They were wild and free and the whole scene blew his mind. Eventually, they let go and out from the house strolled Dave's brother and his lady. They both gave Bob a hug but in a much more gentle fashion than the kids.

"This is my good friend Dave," Bob shared.

Denise moved towards Dave introducing herself, giving him a kiss and a hug. Then it was Sam's turn, and he offered his hand for a shake which somehow then turned into a hug. Dave had not hugged many men – except for when he was drunk – and was a little shocked at first, but then just felt very welcomed. Also, given the set-up, he was sure Sam wasn't a poof. After some chatting and catching up it became clear no one else was staying there at present, and they'd each have a cabin to call their own.

On the way over to their new quarters, they got a good look at the place and Sam was excited to share some new changes with Bob. Sam looked a fair bit older than his brother but you could definitely see the resemblance in their facial features. Sam was very clean cut, especially in comparison with Bob, who had hair past his shoulders and an award-winning beard. At a guess, Sam was about forty five and as for Bob, it was really hard to tell what age he was.

The chicken house had just been redone and it looked good. The chickens seemed happy about it as well and came over to say hello to everyone. The kids called them by their names and poked at them through the wire fence. There were fruit trees everywhere. It was the first time Dave had seen an orange tree in fruit and wandered over to have a closer look.

"Go for it," Denise said. "They are really good this

year and the ones that fall off easily are the ones that are ready to eat."

One dropped straight into Dave's hand as he lightly touched it. *How easy was that*, he thought to himself and began peeling with excitement. As the first piece hit his tongue, it was like an electric shock going through his mouth.

"Wow! Wow! Wow! Amazing!" Dave said, in a blissful manner and kept eating.

The orange was sweet and juicy, a proper vitamin C bomb. His mouth was in heaven and to make it even better, the tree was loaded so he knew it wouldn't be his last.

Sam took his guests over to the cabins and gave Dave the rundown on the wood fire and where everything was. Dave's cabin was beautiful. It was all very simple, yet tidy, clean and luxurious in its own way. It was one big open room, with a huge, comfy-looking bed, a leather couch and there was even an ensuite bathroom, complete with a bathtub that had forest views. Dave felt grateful and thanked Sam endlessly.

Bob and Sam left him to settle in. The afternoon was cooling down and evening wouldn't be too far away. He walked around his new home checking everything out and admiring the simple woodwork and furnishings. This was the first time he'd ever had his own cabin to stay in. He felt like a king and walked out onto the deck which overlooked the orchard, and beyond that, the forest.

Dave was getting cold and decided on a shower. He thoroughly enjoyed the hot water on his shoulders as they were feeling a bit sore from surfing earlier. Those muscles hadn't been used in a long time! His whole body began to melt and relax. He could've stayed in there forever, but he'd been too well drilled in short showers and turned off the tap. As he got out, there was a big, clean, soft towel awaiting him. Next he slipped on the fluffy, white bath robe and giggled to himself looking in the mirror.

"I don't know if I'm a king or a movie star!" he said out loud, throwing some sexy faces at himself.

The fire was already set and all he had to do was light it. It reminded Dave of the slow combustion fire that had been up at the family farm when he was younger. Once that got going it used to heat a big room easily. The flames danced and crackled and he began to fade out heavily. He went and crawled into bed to keep warm, under the big, fluffy doona. It was even more comfortable than it looked and he was asleep in no time.

Just after sunset, Bob came to check in on him, to see how he was going and if he wanted some dinner. When he saw him fast asleep, he slipped away quietly. Bob knew Dave was in need of a lot of rest and that's the reason he'd brought him here. Just to stop, relax and reconnect with the simple things... that was the plan.

Dave didn't wake once during the whole night and eventually woke early the next morning to the sound of a rooster crowing. Outside, the sun had not yet come up but the day was definitely arriving. He looked from his bed, out across the forest to the east, and the sky was filled with an orange radiance. He felt surprised when he remembered he hadn't even had dinner the previous night. Without hesitation, Dave sprung out of bed and put some warm clothes on. He was hungry and went outside to go and see his new friend, the orange tree. The oranges were extremely cold but this didn't stop him from eating a couple. His mouth, exploding with aliveness again.

What a way to start the day, he thought. Dave was keen to investigate the property some more and began to have a look around. He discovered an apple tree and delighted in sampling one.

"This is how it's meant to be," he whispered, with a mouthful. He'd only ever had fruit from the supermarket or the fruit store but it never tasted anything like this.

The start of a bush track winding up the hill caught Dave's eye and he thought a morning walk would be great. It was cold and he wanted to get his body moving. He guessed everyone else was still sleeping and he'd catch up with them later for breakfast. It was quiet. Barely a breath of wind. The trees were dense either side of the track and the ground was a mixture of boggy wet sections and rocky patches. *They've probably had some heavy rain recently*, Dave reasoned, dodging another puddle.

He felt energised from a long sleep and walked quickly up the hill. The clean, fresh, morning air filled his lungs and he felt fantastic. There was a feeling of freedom, of not having to be anywhere at any particular time. The bush began to thin out and there was a clearing up ahead with some large rocks on it. Dave climbed ambitiously to the top. From there he could see the house, the orchard, and further out to the east, the ocean beyond the forest. The sun was beginning to poke its head out of the water, throwing brilliant colours up into the sky. Dave stood there, admiring the spectacular view. The wind was a little stronger now and it cooled his back. All he could hear was the faint cry of the rooster, down towards the house.

He stood there silent, entranced by the rising sun, looking straight into it. For once, no questions filled his mind. A sense of peace... His life had taken a radical turn and he somehow knew it was all for the better.

Dave's stomach began to rumble and he decided to head back down for breakfast. Everyone was up when he arrived and they were all happy to see him. The kids gave him the running hug, for which he was ready this time and then Denise, Sam and even Bob greeted him with a hug. His gay fears were starting to disappear rapidly. It all felt so easy and natural and warmed his heart. Breakfast was laid out on a huge wooden table. It consisted of a big pot of porridge, a bowl of fruit, bread and an assortment of interesting-looking spreads.

Everyone sat down and joined hands before eating. This made Dave a touch uncomfortable but he was open to it. He wondered if they were religious and it was a sort of church thing. Sam began to speak:

"Thank you Mother Earth for providing us with this beautiful food. Thank you for our good health, our abundance, our joy and for bringing these two amazing men into our home. Yaaahhooooo!" he cried out and then began to laugh loudly in a similar style to Bob which triggered everyone at the table to join in. This threw a bit of a twist on Dave putting them in the church box and he no longer knew what to think. They definitely never used to be that loose at Sunday School! He hooked into a big bowl of steaming hot porridge, complete with nuts, seeds and berries. It was delicious.

Over breakfast they discussed how Bob and Dave could help out around the place. It was decided that three or four hours each day in exchange for food and shelter was a fair deal. This excited Dave as he was very eager to learn about looking after fruit trees and growing vegetables.

The job for the morning was to pull out weeds around the base of the trees and then put mulch down. This was a rich combination of straw, compost and seaweed. Dave enjoyed the work but as the morning went on, his energy started fading out and he wasn't feeling so good. They stopped for lunch, which consisted of fresh salad from the garden, with roasted sweet potato that Denise had cooked. Unfortunately, Dave didn't have too much of a chance to get excited about it. He could hardly keep awake. He ate half his plate and went back to the cabin for a shower and a lie down.

The bed was even more comfortable than he had

remembered from the night before and again, he was asleep in seconds. Dave slept… and slept… and slept… not waking up for dinner for the second night in a row. He awoke to the sound of the rooster crowing and hardly knew where he was. He must have slept for fifteen or sixteen hours. It was bizarre – he had never slept this much in his whole life.

Dave was ravenous and headed straight out to the fruit trees. It was a similar morning to the one before and he was actually feeling really good again. This whole up and down energy thing was getting to him and he felt guilty for sleeping so much. He wished he could've helped out more with the gardening and been a bit more social. He was a visitor and all he was doing was sleeping. After a feed of oranges and apples, he walked back up the hill to take in the sunrise.

"Morning Dave," Sam said, with a big smile on his face. Opening up the door into the kitchen and sharing a hug. "You had another good sleep, hey."

"Yeah, fourteen hours or somethin', don't know what's goin' on with that." Dave said, looking at the ground. "Sorry for missin' dinner again."

"No need for an apology there. Bob was saying you've been through a rough patch lately."

"Yeah, pretty much."

Sam lifted himself up, taking a seat on the bench and caught Dave's eye: "Would you like to know how I ended up out here in the wilderness?"

"Yeah, love to."

"After fifteen years working in the LA finance

industry, I was fairly well cooked you might say. My wife had taken off, my health was in danger... I was an unhappy man. I thought I was doing well but in the end, it all got the better of me." Sam caught Dave's eye again. "There's some similarities to your story but I didn't catch it early enough... Anyway, one morning at the cafe I spotted a little flyer on the window, advertising a life coach. I had always been way to stubborn to follow a road like that, but it grabbed me. I was desperate. Can't remember what was written on there... but I called her up and after three months my world was transformed. Probably had something to do with me falling in love with the coach too!"

"You serious?" Dave laughed.

"Yeah, Denise was the coach."

"No way!"

"Wild hey... Next I quit my job, started dating the coach, had a good rest and then went travelling around the world with her. Eventually we ended up here."

Sam now worked as a financial consultant two days per week from home, which was a much better balance. Many of the people who stayed in their cabins were from Sydney and totally inspired by Sam and Denise's story and the way they lived. Often, the guests would leave with a new outlook on their lives. It was a very positive set-up; the retreat was all about slowing life down and letting the nervous system unwind itself from the madness of modern day life.

After hearing all this, Dave realised everything was perfectly okay. As Bob had said, this was exactly what the doctor ordered. He breathed out with a huge sigh of relief.

"Thanks Sam, I'm startin' to get it. For so long I've been pushin' myself and tryin' to find out what's wrong, when all I probably need to do is just slow down. Life's been pretty crazy lately and I'm glad to be here. Don't know if I've ever allowed myself to relax so much."

"My pleasure Dave. That's why we set this place up – a place where you can step out of the rat race, stop and rest. We're not robots you know, we're human beings. What's the big rush anyway?" Sam laughed, "that's not what I used to think though! Make yourself right at home here and rest as much as you need. You're young and healthy. You'll come back into balance in no time."

"Yeah, thanks Sam. I really appreciate it. I feel at home here."

The next four or five days became a routine of waking early, drinking two big glasses of fresh spring water, eating fruit, walking up the hill and then having a hearty breakfast with the family. Dave would then help out around the place for the morning doing various jobs which he loved. Lunch would be served and then he would head back to his cabin to rest and read. Sleep would soon follow and most evenings he continued to miss dinner and sleep right through. He was regularly sleeping between ten and sixteen hours each day and was slowly but surely beginning to feel better.

There was a large bookcase in his room filled

with some very interesting books. He figured they must've been Denise's, as many of them were about life coaching and self-development. As he read bits and pieces from the varied assortment, he began to see the bigger picture of his life and it brought him a sense of relief. He realised he wasn't such a head case after all. One key message he gained was that life gives you whatever you focus on. He could see the pattern of his last few months, where all he thought about was his broken heart and how sick he was, and things hadn't changed much.

One morning, as he was standing on the rocks at the top of the hill taking in the sunrise, he made a decision that he would now focus on the positive things about his health and his girlfriend leaving. He realised that he had enough energy to climb the hill and garden every morning. That made him feel good about himself. He also realised that he was only nineteen and his whole life lay before him. It was probably a blessing Anne was off in Europe enjoying herself. Dave thought of all the other beautiful girls in the world that he was yet to meet and a spark of joy shot through his body.

As he strolled back towards the house for breakfast, the awareness came that something else had changed today. He felt a different sort of energy moving through him. He'd slowed down a lot and the energy he now embodied felt more grounded, with a quiet strength about it. The previous mornings he'd had this excitable, wanting-to-do-something vibe. Today however, he was energised but relaxed at the same time.

5. PANCAKE EYES

Dave was a little behind schedule this morning and when he got to the house, breakfast was well under way. He was really starting to enjoy the morning hugs from everyone and hugging back just as warmly. He was hungry, as usual, and his big bowl of porridge vanished before his eyes. The sun was shining and it was a magic morning. The full team, including the kids, were on the gardening program today.

Denise and Dave teamed up to weed one of the many veggie gardens. The one they chose contained kale, broccoli and a huge selection of what Dave thought were lettuce.

"Is this all lettuce?" he asked, sweeping his hand out in front of him.

"Yes Dave. We are very passionate about growing

as much variety as possible, especially in our fresh greens. We've got oak leaf, *lollo rosso*, rocket," Denise said, pointing out each one and revealing a dozen names that were new to Dave's ears. "We manage to source heirloom seeds, from a local old farmer down the road."

"What do you mean, heirloom seeds?" Dave enquired, frothing to learn more.

"Well, my understanding is that these days it's very important to know where your seeds come from." Denise took a seat on the edge of the garden bed. "The heirloom seeds are just a fancy name for the original variety of seeds that haven't been manipulated or genetically modified. They've been passed down through the generations. There's a debate raging over the impact that GMO – genetically modified – seeds and crops are having on the environment and people's health."

Dave jumped in: "Yeah, I've seen that on tele, on some current affairs show... didn't give it much attention though."

"Well, it's a no brainer," she said strongly, shaking her head. "The only benefit of GMO seed and crops is to the large multi-national companies who are using them to take control of the worlds food supply. It's a dangerous practice that threatens the entire eco-system. It's really frightening!" Denise finished, with a concerned look on her face.

Dave was a little confused. "Why do you need to modify nature when it seems to work perfectly already?" he questioned, trying to understand the whole concept and why anyone would want to take control of the worlds food supply? It seemed like something from a movie... Not a kids movie though!

"I hear you Dave and that's another part of the reason we moved here. To regain some control over our lives and what we put in our kids' mouths. It's such a blessing to have fresh, home grown fruit and veggies. Half the things in the supermarket these days, you really have no idea what's in them or what's been done to the ingredients beforehand. Unfortunately, most people are so busy they don't have time to study those things and their health suffers. It's actually quite sad."

She stood up and gave her hands a good shake. "I need to watch I don't get too caught up in it all though, because I end up feeling awful myself and that's no good for anyone. Especially me." Denise was now shaking her whole body and making a few powerful breathing sounds. It looked awfully similar to one of Bob's moves. Dave wondered what this shaking thing was all about. "Aaaaaahhhhhh... that's much better," she said, breathing out with relief. "With these sorts of things happening on the planet, it takes constant awareness to stay positive and energised. If we are going to create a better world, we need to focus on just how good life really is and how we can make it even better!"

Denise was now looking much more alive and Dave felt inspired by her words.

"It's funny you say that, 'cause the books I've been readin' in the cabin have all been pointin' to the fact that you create your own world by what you focus on, and I'm fully startin' to get it."

Denise was amazed with his insight and very happy he'd been reading her books. She told him, that if he could get a handle on thinking good-feeling thoughts most of the time, his life would continue to evolve in a positive direction. She was very interested in Dave's journey and where he was headed.

"What do you want for your life, Dave?" she asked, pulling out a weed.

"Dunno really. I've been askin' that question a bit lately and have absolutely no idea to be honest. One thing I do know is that I wanna be healthy and have my energy back."

"Why is it, that you want to be healthy and have more energy?" she enquired.

"Well, when I'm healthy, energised and clear, I'm heaps better at makin' good decisions for my life. I feel like I've been in a fog for months. Since being here though, I'm gettin' clearer and clearer each day."

"Great to hear. This truly is a magical place and it has transformed both Sam and my lives dramatically. We were both totally different people ten years ago." Denise was now standing closer to Dave with the morning sun on her face. Like the kids, she also had a sparkle in her eyes and was very healthy looking. "A question that I love asking some of my clients in the early stages of our work together, is what would they do with their lives if they won ten million dollars today? It's a creative way of opening up to more choice and possibility. Money is a fantastic one to start with as well, because so often it's used as an excuse to stay stuck... So, tell me Dave, what is it that you'd do if you won ten million dollars today?"

The question stunned Dave a bit and he stood up straight, throwing a big bunch of weeds into the bucket. He'd talked about winning Lotto before but never really thought what he'd do with the money. Ten million was a lot! What would he do? How would his life change?

"Far out Denise, I have no idea what I'd do," he answered, defeated.

"That's okay," Denise said, in a caring tone. "It catches a lot of people off guard. It's a great one to think about though, because if you want your life to be different in some ways, it helps a lot to start visualising it and feeling how you'd like it to be."

Dave didn't quite understand or fully hear Denise. He was still stuck on the question and the options of what he'd do with ten million dollars. How much would he give away to his family and friends? Would he travel the world? He could even organise a surf trip with all of his mates and pay for the lot. What sort of car would he get? Was he ready to buy a house? Question after question and possibility after possibility ran wild through his mind.

Denise could see he was struggling with it all.

"Probably best to just take one step at a time right now and focus on yourself being healthy, energised and clear. Please Dave, utilise this place to rest and enjoy the simple gifts life has to offer. Fresh air, sunshine, healthy food, relaxation and good sleep. It will do wonders for you. And, the truth is, you don't even need ten million dollars for these things," she ended, with a light giggle.

"Yeah, one step at a time's good. I'm definitely startin' to feel better and better each day though. Thanks Denise."

Dave was weeding in amongst the broccoli now and asked if it could be included with lunch. It was dark green and just bursting with goodness. It was as if his body was talking with him and asking for it. Denise agreed and revealed the lunch plan with Dave. The mid-morning sun warmed his back and he continued on with the gardening program, until the whole bed was done and it looked a million dollars… or should it be ten million dollars!

The kids were playing chasings around the garden and having an absolute ball. They were so energised and natural, Dave had not once seen them during the day playing computer games or vegging out inside. They loved to be out in the fresh air, running around, kicking the ball, chasing each other or helping out the grown ups. Spontaneously, Dave joined in the chasing and the kids loved it. Once he'd caught them, they then turned on him. It was an awesome sight as Dave weaved in and out of the fruit trees to get away. They giggled and ran and giggled some more, till the three of them fell down on the grass, exhausted. Dave felt like a kid again – so alive and free!

A little later, lunch was served and the lightly steamed broccoli was exactly what he needed.

Combined with some brown rice and fresh local fish, it all hit the spot perfectly. Since being there, he'd eaten the healthiest, most wholesome meals he'd ever had. He felt extremely nourished and wasn't getting the in-between-meal sweet cravings he usually got. Fruit straight off the trees and vegetables of all description, fresh from the garden. What a way to live. It all seemed so easy and so right.

It turned out, that Bob had been keeping an eye on the surf report and the following morning was shaping up to be real good. Sitting out on the grass, having a cuppa after lunch, a plan was pieced together. Apparently, a reef break fifteen minutes down the road would be pumping. It was Sam's favourite surf spot, so he decided on joining the operation. It was agreed they'd leave shortly after the rooster crowed the following morning.

Dave slept well and woke to his new alarm clock. This morning's routine would be different from the previous ones. Out of habit he headed straight for the orange tree but wasn't all that hungry and decided to save the fruit for later. He also grabbed a few extras for the lads. The four wheel drive was packed with boards and wetsuits and off they drove into the cool autumn morning.

On the way there, Bob and Sam reminisced about this particular surf spot and how they'd had some epic sessions there over the years. They even shared some of their Californian childhood surf stories, which really got the laughter flowing. Dave had not surfed many reef breaks and was excited at the prospect. They turned off down a dirt track. It was a bumpy old road and Dave understood why they'd taken the four wheel drive.

"Well, here we are," Sam said, as they pulled up on top of a headland overlooking a big bay. In the northern corner was the reef break. "It's not as big as I'd hoped," he continued, "but it's still pumping."

Bob was like a teenager. Totally frothing and couldn't sit still. He looked back at Dave. "Man, you're gunna love this joint. Lets get out there!"

It was actually hard to tell just how big it was, 'cause they were quite high up above the ocean. The wave was a peak, with a short right breaking back towards the rocks and a long left rattling off in the other direction. There wasn't another soul in sight and the surf team eagerly pulled their wetsuits on. It was a cold morning with a stiff off-shore breeze and the sun was only just out of the ocean.

They steadily made their way down a goat track towards the water, stopping every now and then to watch a wave or two exploding on the reef. Both the brothers were hooting and screaming like crazy kids while Dave was a little more reserved and studying the waves as best he could. Once they got to ocean level, Dave could see just how amazing this place was. It was a perfect reef set-up with potential for a good tube ride in both directions. Sam had said it wasn't all that big from the top, but now Dave could see clearly what was going on… and it looked solid, easily bigger than the ceiling in his bedroom. He'd surfed waves this size before but never over a reef. He was up for the challenge though and feeling really good.

Sam and Bob jumped from the rocks into the cool green ocean and Dave wasn't far behind. The three of them paddled out in a rip running alongside the rocks. They arrived at the peak without even getting their hair wet. A wave rolled in and Sam was in exactly the right position. Bob hooted loudly as he paddled into it. "Go Sam… yoooooooohhhhhh!" Sam went left and Dave watched from behind as the wave peeled for over fifty metres, before he saw him flicking off the back of it, with his arms up in the air, yelling and screaming.

The next two contenders waited patiently for the ocean to produce some more of its gifts. Bob was always super relaxed in the water and as soon as the next wave came in, he said: "Okay Dave, this one's all yours!" Dave began paddling and getting himself into the best spot. The swell reared up behind him and he stroked like a mad-man, half excited and half freaking out.

He felt the tail of his board begin to lift… he was on. All he could see metres below him was a big, black, shallow reef and this completely freaked him out. For a second he hesitated and went to pull back, but it was far too late for that… The wave had him firmly in its clutches and all he could do now was to go into full-on survival mode and prepare for the worst. Suddenly, it seemed much bigger than he'd thought… He managed to push his board aside as the wave tossed him into the air like a piece of driftwood. He was now at the total mercy of Mother Ocean. Dave slammed onto the flat water at the base of the wave, the impact squeezing all the air out of his body in a second. The liquid wrecking ball followed shortly behind, driving him underwater and shaking him to pieces, like a rag doll in the mouth of a pit bull. There was a sharp thump on his right knee as he hit the reef. He'd never experienced anything like it... It was the washing machine from hell!

Panic began to set in as Dave realised he needed air sooner than later, and he opened his eyes to get some idea of where he was. By now the major turbulence had passed and he scrambled for the light in survival mode, adrenalin coursing through his body at warp speed. He broke through the surface gasping for breath, with eyes as wide as pancakes and his heart beating a million miles per hour. He grabbed a quick half breath before being mown down by the next wave. This was getting serious... Luckily he'd been washed in quite a way now and the intensity of the whitewater was much, much less. He made a mad scramble for the surface again and burst through the foam taking a huge, well-needed breath. The next couple of waves washed over him ferociously but they were nothing compared to the first two.

Dave felt like he'd just done a round with Mohamed Ali and was completely ruined. He was alive, but barely even knew where he was or what was going on.

"You alright dude?" came a sharp voice, followed quickly by a hand grabbing him and lifting him slightly out of the water. It was Sam and he'd seen the whole thing. "That was one of the best wipe-outs I've seen for a long while!" he said, with a wild laugh, relieved that Dave hadn't drowned. "Are you okay mate?" he continued more seriously, realising Dave wasn't in the best shape and looked as white as a cuttle fish.

"Yeah. That was heavy man!" Dave replied, in a somewhat bewildered voice, still gasping for breath... "I banged my knee pretty hard on the bottom, think my wetsuit saved me though... it's just aching a bit. Wow, that was heavy!"

At that moment they heard a loud hoot and both turned to see Bob dropping into a beautiful looking wave. It was even bigger than Dave's one and with the morning sun behind it, the colours were phenomenal; Greens, oranges and even yellows dancing through the roof. Bob looked like he'd done it a thousand times before. He was ultra relaxed and in perfect sync with the ocean. He made it all look so effortless.

After a slow, drawn-out bottom turn he eased his way up into the tubing part of the wave. He then disappeared and both Sam and Dave were hooting so loudly that Dave forgot all about his throbbing knee for a second. The wave continued to break down the reef, for a moment Bob appeared and then vanished again deep into the tube. The lads were now silent, totally blown away with the wave, hoping he would make it. Suddenly Bob came flying out with his hands above his head, screaming ecstatically and cracking up at the same time. It was like watching a surf movie. Dave had no idea Bob was such a competent surfer.

For the next hour the brothers continued surfing while Dave went in and sat on the beach, watching the whole show unfold. They were both exceptional surfers and continued to get wave after wave and only fell a couple of times each in the whole session. This reef break surfing was next level and Dave had lots to learn and many fears to overcome. He'd found a spot on the beach out of the cool off-shore breeze and the morning sun was keeping him warm. There was still no one around for miles and Dave couldn't believe it. If this was the city it would have been packed. His knee hurt but he felt relaxed, content and happy to be alive.

This last week and a bit had really changed something within him. Something had settled. He hadn't thought much at all about Anne and his broken heart. Hadn't taken any of his medicine. Hadn't checked his phone… well, he didn't even have 'em with him! A lot of those things didn't seem to matter much any more.

It was such a blessing that he had the time, space and support to listen to his body. Rather than seeing sleeping all day as wrong, or not tough, he now had a new appreciation of how healing it can actually be. He could see how most people weren't giving themselves a chance to listen to their bodies and to stop and rest when they needed to.

The knowledge he'd picked up about living simply and more sustainably in the country was inspiring. Imagine, if everyone had the opportunity to walk outside in the morning and pick a piece of fresh fruit from the tree. Dave was sure that the abundance of vital, alive fruit and veggies was part of the reason that he was feeling so much healthier. Also, the spring water he'd been drinking was apparently loaded with goodies too. He couldn't wait to get back up to the car for his morning orange.

Sam and Bob eventually came in and gave each other a huge hug on the beach. It turned out it'd been over a year since they'd had such quality, uncrowded surf together. They were both super stoked.

"How you goin' Dave?" Bob asked, "I heard you got annihilated on that wave!"

"Yeah… best ever wipeout I reckon. I'm fine now, was a good wake-up call though. I've got lots to learn about surfing reef breaks and by the looks of it, you can both be my teachers!"

Everyone laughed and they headed back up the steep, rocky path to the car. The morning sun was now much warmer and really lighting up the day. Dave's knee was feeling better too. As soon as they arrived at the car, he grabbed an orange and peeled it, sharing it with the surf team. They all stood there overlooking the ocean, enjoying the fruit.

"How does it get any better than this?" Bob asked, with a huge smile on his face. Just as he finished, a pod of dolphins swam through where they'd been surfing. There must've been at least ten of them and they all rode one wave together… The true masters of surfing! So skilful, jumping, diving and fully enjoying themselves. It was a sight to behold. The three men stood there dumbstruck, with their mouths full of juicy orange.

6. THE GREEN WORM

On the drive back home, Sam took a detour through town to stop at the local organic fruit and veggie store. He shared with Bob and Dave that tomorrow he would be starting his monthly two day juice fast and needed a few extra bits and pieces they weren't growing. Since getting his health back on track years ago, he'd kept up this routine every month and his overall well-being had benefited greatly from it.

"What actually is a juice fast?" Dave asked, inquisitively.

"Basically, it's just living on fresh fruit and veggie juice and nothing else. This gives your body a rest from constantly digesting food and uses that spare energy to heal and balance your system. It's simple and very effective."

"So for two whole days, all you have is juice," Dave questioned, blown away with the idea.

"Yes, that's right. It sounds a little insane, but once you've experienced it, you soon realise it's definitely not. The amount of work our bodies do, digesting food twenty four hours a day is overwhelming. I'd never really stopped to think about it, before I began fasting. I've got a whole new perspective now. I'm also much more aware of what I put in my mouth, especially the quantity!"

"Do ya reckon it'd be good for me?"

"No doubt. You've already started with the no-dinner fast," laughed Sam. "I would recommend it to you for sure. Your body seems to be undergoing some healing at the moment, and this will only benefit the process."

"Righto, I'm in. I'd love to join if that's okay."

"Sure thing Dave. You can always give it a shot as well, and if for some reason your not enjoying it, you just stop. Like I said, it's simple."

A big smile appeared on Bob's face. "Man, I'm not one to miss out on a juice fast," he said, leaning back and giving Dave a high five. "I'm in too!"

"Fantastic. The more the merrier. It could be a lot of fun if we all do it together. Denise usually joins in too." Sam said.

You could feel the excitement in the car. An epic morning's surfing, dolphins and now plans for a team juice fast! Dave was intrigued and sensed his body would benefit a lot from the process. Town was quiet this morning and they parked right outside the store. Dave would finally get to check out an organic fruit and veggie shop. He still had no real idea of what the difference was, or what all the hype was about, but he was keen to get inside and see.

From the outside it didn't look like much but once he opened the door, a whole new world was revealed. He was greeted by boxes of potatoes that were still covered in dirt, carrots that still had green tops and large beetroots, with big stalks and leaves hanging off them. Most of the fruit and veg you would normally find at the supermarket was there, but it all looked very different. The produce was various shapes and sizes and he even saw a spinach leaf with a big, green worm on it. He called Bob over and showed him, with a laugh: "So what's this whole organic thing about Bob? Denise schooled me yesterday about genetically modified food, but I still don't fully get it?"

"Well, I reckon that worm answers the question perfectly. If it's good enough for a worm to eat, it means it's good enough for us to eat! The basic deal is man, organic farming has been practised for hundreds of years and it simply means growin' food without chemical growth enhancement or poison to keep the insects off it. Organic produce is also far more nutritious 'cause it grows more slowly in rich, alive, natural soil. Also the GMO crops that Denise was talkin' about are so drenched in poisonous herbicides and pesticides that it's killin' bees, birds and who knows what else?

"Unfortunately man, these days in big business, it's all about maximisin' production and profits at the expense of the consumer's health. That's why it's so important for us to support the organic growers because ultimately, it's about the health of the people and the health of the planet. Does that make sense?"

"Yeah, I totally get it Bob, and I now understand why I've never seen a worm on the veggies at the supermarket. What I don't get, is why would people buy fruit and veggies they knew were sprayed with poison?"

"I don't get that either man, and a lot of the time I'm guessin' that people don't know. They just assume it's okay, 'cause everyone's doin' it. It's nuts! But the cool thing is though, it's changin' and the organic movement is growin' quickly. It's all about education and awareness."

Sam had a huge basket, already loaded with a colourful selection of goodies for the team's juicing adventure. The pretty girl behind the counter started weighing up the fruit and veg, stacking it neatly into a cardboard box. Dave was still only a few steps inside the shop and had so much more to discover. He knew Sam would be done in a few minutes and felt an urgency to take in as much as he could in a short time.

There was a section of bulk foods, such as rice, nuts and seeds. An area of shelving which contained various vitamins and protein powders. They even had organic shampoos and what truly flipped Dave out was they had an all-natural, organic sunscreen! A whole new world was continuing to open up for him and it was exciting. The lads were already out at the car and he didn't want to keep them waiting.

"Thanks, I love your shop!" Dave said to the cute girl working there, as he hurried out the door.

"My pleasure. Enjoy your day," she replied with a smile.

Once back in the car, Bob handed Dave a small brown paper bag. "Try this, it's awesome!" he shared, just knowing Dave would love it.

"Thanks mate." Dave wasted no time in investigating the gift. It was a sweet little ball, made up of nuts, dried fruit and coconut flakes. He savoured each mouthful, trying to decipher every ingredient. It was healthy food and it tasted great. The biscuit jar at the hardware store would never be the same again!

After such an action-packed morning, the three of them were ravenous for a good, solid breakfast and once home, created a scrambled-eggs-on-toast feast. The homemade bread Denise had baked just set the meal off and everyone was content. Sam cranked up some classic, relaxing music and the whole family, including the kids, went outside and sat on the grass in the morning sun. It was the perfect autumn day and the property looked very neat and cared for. The work they'd all done over the past few weeks had fully transformed FOR REST ECO RETREAT and Dave felt proud to see it there before him. The kids played and wrestled on the grass while the rest of them enjoyed their tea.

It turned out today was house cleaning day and the cabins (as well as the main house) would get a good going over. Dave was feeling a little tired after the big breakfast. His morning adrenalin rush had also well and truly worn off. He recounted his wipeout and just how close he'd been to drowning. It was for sure the gnarliest one he'd ever had. He felt a renewed sense of how happy he was to be alive, sitting there in the sun with a hot cuppa. *It's interesting how a near-death experience can give you a new outlook on life*, he thought and then jumped to his feet: "Okay, I'm ready for action. Where do I find the cleaning gear?" he asked enthusiastically, while throwing a few karate moves at the kids who were still playing on the lawn. They responded by attacking him and wrestling him down to the ground.

"All the basic cleaning gear is in the bathroom cupboard in each cabin. We've got the vacuum and mops here in the main house. You guys concentrate on the cabins first and once you're done you can come and give us a hand," Sam said, in a relaxed, assertive way.

Bob and Dave headed back to their cabins and Dave went straight in to find the cleaning gear. All he could find in the cupboard was a bucket, a bottle of vinegar and some bi-carb soda. He was sure he'd heard the instructions clearly and kept on looking. After finding nothing else he went outside to call Bob from his verandah.

"Hey Bob, I can't seem to find the cleanin' gear. All I've found is cookin' stuff. Did you find any?"

"Yeah, I've just found the basics though. Vinegar, bi-carb, eucalyptus oil and some rags."

"You mean that stuff's the cleaning gear?" Dave questioned, a touch confused.

"Sure man, they live chemical-free here, and use these simple things you'd normally find in the kitchen for cleaning."

"Do they work?" he asked, not believing it to be possible.

"Too right, they actually work well and it's much healthier for us and Mother Earth too."

Dave thought for a minute and remembered when he was cleaning his shower back at home. The fumes from the mould killer spray would make him dizzy and feel sick. He used to hate that part. There was so much new information coming to him. He was soaking it all up like a sponge. It was inspiring to be around people who were living differently than he was used to. He went over to Bob's cabin to question him on this new technique.

Bob showed Dave how to fill the little spray bottle with water, vinegar and a few drops of eucalyptus oil. He looked like a mad scientist making up a potion and then went into full acting mode, displaying his cleaning technique. It was hilarious.

"You spray a bit here, you spray a bit there," Bob began in some strange, German-sounding accent. "Give it a good rub with the rag… like so, and for these tough little stains in the shower, you sprinkle a light dusting of this magical powder. Then give it a good scrub."

Dave was in stitches by this point and Bob couldn't help himself either. The two of them laughed and laughed and when Bob took a few spare breaths he continued the act, and then laughed some more.

It was a lively start to Dave's chemical-free cleaning experience and to top it off, he didn't have a headache from toxic fumes!

Dave learnt plenty from Bob, Sam and Denise about the simplicity and health benefits of chemical-free cleaning. Again, he just couldn't understand why so many more people didn't know about these things. Once he got his head around it, it all made so much sense. In a couple of weeks, the knowledge he'd gained about the simple things in life had changed his world. Sleeping, eating and cleaning would never be the same again.

The last job for the day was to go and help Sam refill the water bottles from a spring at the back of the property. Sam explained that during the juice fast it was important to drink loads of water and as the supply was down, it was time to get some more. They loaded half a dozen water containers into the four wheel drive and drove up a track behind the house. Sam explained that part of the reason he'd purchased the property was because of the spring. During his health turnaround, he'd madly researched all the things he could do to bring his body back into balance. One of the key pieces he discovered, was the profound benefits of good quality drinking water.

"It's vital and it's overlooked by so many," Sam said. "There is tonnes of misinformation. Some people think tap water is fine, others think rain water is the best. But from all my research, unpolluted spring water came up as the winner. There is just so much life in it! It also makes sense because that is what humans originally drank. We have a huge National Park behind us here, so there is no pollution from farming or industry that effects the water. I've even had it tested. It's clean and jam packed with the right balance of minerals."

"Well, I've certainly been enjoyin' it," Dave shared, joining Sam's excitement.

The road was rough and the day was drawing to a close. Dave was almost on information overload, his head feeling tight. He'd caught most of what Sam had said and was looking forward to seeing the spring. The car came to a stop at the base of a small, rocky hill. Out to the west, the sun was sinking behind the mountains. They both jumped out to take in the scene. It was magnificent. In the distance a bunch of kookaburras were singing in the sunset.

They grabbed a few containers each and Dave followed Sam over to an area he had not spotted from the car. There was a thick cluster of green trees which huddled around the entrance to a small cave. The fading light made it hard to see what was down there. Sam took the lead, with Dave close behind. It wasn't a huge cave but the temperature was definitely cooler and it was ultra-quiet, all except for the trickling noise of water.

Dave could see the water pouring from the rock face. A short copper pipe had been jammed in there, making it easier to fill the bottles. It was surreal! The water poured out onto the rocks below and was then channelled for a couple of metres, before disappearing again into the earth. Dave put his mouth to the fountain for a drink. It was cold, refreshing and almost tasted bubbly. He ended up using his hands as a bowl, finding it a bit easier to drink that way. What an experience. To drink water coming straight from the earth! They filled all the containers, by which time night had fully arrived.

Back at the house, everyone agreed to have a light dinner of steamed veggies only, in preparation for the next two days. Tonight, more than ever, Dave felt like part of the family. He'd been busy helping out most of the day and he'd definitely earned his steamed veggies. Amazingly, his energy had remained fairly steady all day, but he knew an early night was necessary and he also knew, he would sleep really, really well.

The night was chaotic, filled with heavy showers, wind and thunderstorms. The rain continued on through the morning and it was so heavy that Dave didn't even hear the alarm clock go off.

7. PIPE CLEAN

"First juice is up Dave!" came a loud scream from Bob, through the noise of the rain on the roof.

"Be there in a minute!" Dave yelled back, hoping Bob would hear. He was starving hungry by now, especially after last night's steamed veggies entrée. He'd even been hungry by the time he went to bed. *This could be a long two days*, he thought, getting out of bed and putting on some warm clothes.

His cabin looked beautiful this morning. Everything was put away neatly and the whole place was spotlessly clean. A slight scent of eucalyptus oil was still in the air. It felt good to wake up in a clean room. He was so used to leaving his clothes all over the floor and this morning he appreciated the difference.

A quick run through the rain and he met everyone

in the kitchen, already half way through their juices. A choir of good mornings filled the air and the usual chain of warm hugs came Dave's way. Even the kids joined in today, sharing a big hug with Dave – one at a time though, in a more traditional manner. The big juicer was set up on the bench next to a cutting board and by the looks of it, the production line had been in full swing. Denise handed Dave a large glass of purple, thick liquid with orange foam on top.

"Thanks… Cheers!" he responded, receiving the glass and holding it up in the air. It reminded him of a scene in the pub one night when he and his mates were all on the black beer. He took the glass to his lips and cautiously poured in the first sip. The juice was dense and heavy with a powerful kick of ginger. It was actually far better than it looked.

"That's beautiful. I was a bit hesitant 'cause it looks wild, but I'm into it now, thanks," he said, taking another sip.

"Really good to drink it slowly," Bob shared, sounding calm as usual. "I heard a teacher once say to eat your liquid and drink your food. Especially these next few days, if you drink your juice slowly, your body will get a lot more out of it."

Sam had the fire cranked up and it was extremely cosy inside. The rain and wind continued to hammer and the lads shared some surf stories from the day before with Denise and the kids.

"Feels like winter may come early this year," Sam said, looking across at Bob. "Are you going to the desert again?"

"Sure bro, I'm ready to go back. We'll take off later this week. Man, I just know Dave's gunna love it there. I pulled the pin on my job at the movie store, so I'm free as a bird. What do ya reckon Dave?"

Dave was taken by surprise. He hadn't thought of going anywhere. He was really starting to settle in and love it where he was right now. As soon as Bob mentioned the movie store, it had put him in a spin. Shit… He hadn't even phoned his parents! They must be worried sick! What about his work? He knew Bob had sorted it, but it'd almost been two weeks. Did they know how long he'd be gone?

"Geez… I just thought about my parents. They must be really worried. Is it okay if I give 'em a call Sam?"

"Sure, no problem. You can use the phone in my office."

"Thanks," Dave said, and headed straight there in a mild panic.

It rang for ages and was finally picked up by the answering machine. The recording of his Mum's voice sounded different… he hardly even recognised her. He left a clear message explaining he was all good and apologised for taking so long to call. He hadn't even thought about his family once since arriving there, and felt guilty for it. He wondered why no one had been home, wondered how they all were. It was strange. He missed them, but didn't feel the need to see 'em.

Dave just sat there in Sam's office chair, sipping away at his purple juice. He'd become attached to the comfort of his new home and didn't feel all that good about the prospect of leaving. He'd also just heard that the following weekend the cabins were booked and they'd have to hit the road anyway. He'd miss his new found paradise. The way these people lived was simple, healthy and relaxed. Dave knew deep inside that's how he wanted to live.

Back in the kitchen everyone was interested to see how he'd made out with his parents and if everything was okay. He told them that he'd got the answering machine and how he couldn't believe how he'd almost forgotten about his family.

"Relax," Denise shared, in a soothing manner. "You've been asleep for most of that time, remember!" which brought a laugh to the gang. Dave felt lighter and a little more able to see the bigger picture. Sam reached out, giving Dave a glass of spring water:

"Chase your juice down with this. It will help to clean the pipes."

"Cool, thanks. I really appreciate the help you've all given me these past couple of weeks. I haven't felt this good in months."

Dave put down his water and felt the need to give everyone a hug, starting with Sam. As he was hugging him, Denise jumped in also, hugging them both. Bob couldn't resist and joined in as well. The kids saw what was happening from the other side of the room and raced across, giggling. "Team hug!" they screamed, hitting the huddle of bodies at speed.

Dave was now in the middle of the biggest hug he'd ever experienced. Initially his mind was busy, questioning just what the hell was going on, eventually something let go and his body totally relaxed. Mind went quiet. Tears began sliding down his cheeks and onto Sam's shoulder. *Oh no... here we go again*, he thought, before melting into the warmhearted people surrounding him.

He could've just stayed there forever. The tears continued to flow and he was okay with that, especially now he knew it was tough to cry. The biggest hug ever slowly unravelled and Dave decided not to hide his warrior tears.

"Luckily I'm drinkin' heaps of water," he said quietly, a smirk appearing on his face. "'Cause if the tears keep comin' at this rate, I'll be dehydrated before I know it."

They all laughed together, while Dave continued to laugh and cry at the same time. Bob came over and gave him another hug of reassurance. Pulling away, he looked softly at Dave.

"So... what do ya reckon little bro? Ready for another adventure?" Dave looked him straight in the eyes and smiled.

"Yeah... I'm ready," he replied, as another sparkling tear fell from the corner of his left eye.

The storms continued to rumble for hours and only began clearing in the late afternoon. The day was spent in front of the fire, planning the next mission. A big map of the country was spread out on the floor. Excitement was in the air. Sam and Denise gave tips and insights from their travels, while Bob gave the rundown on specific surf spots and the desert camp, which was to be their final destination. It was a monstrous drive but from the description Bob gave of the place, it was well and truly worth it.

Dave was frothing about the proposed adventure, but as the afternoon progressed, he realised the distance and time involved and began to question the whole thing. Would the $240 left in the kitty, plus his $400 be enough? Was he out of his mind joining such a grand adventure with only enough money for a few weeks? What about his job at the hardware? Would he be letting the team down?

His head began to ache and he had this weird chemical taste in his mouth. The only thing he'd eaten all day… well, he hadn't eaten anything! All he'd had, were two peculiar-looking juices and several glasses of water. Dave was beginning to feel very average.

"I'm not sure what's going on but I've got this horrid taste in my mouth and I'm gettin' a headache," he said, in a wobbly sort of voice. "It's strange… It's just been slowly gettin' worse for a little while now."

"This is great!" Sam shared passionately. "It used to happen to me all the time. When you start doing these juice fasts, it gives your system such a rest, that it actually has time and energy to start getting rid of toxins and garbage in your body that have been sitting there for years. All sorts of weird and wonderful things can happen, but see it as a good thing if you can.

"Also, detoxing too much too soon is not a good thing, so it's really important to listen to your body. A mild cleansing reaction like this is fine though. Take it easy and keep drinking water to help flush it all out."

Dave had trouble grasping the whole concept. "You mean it's a good thing that I'm feelin' so shitty?"

"It took me a while to get it as well but these days I rarely feel crap because I've removed so many toxins already. Our bodies are superb creations and can perform miracles, given the right conditions," Sam continued in an inspiring voice.

Dave instantly felt a little better, understanding now what was happening and his mind expanded some more. *Imagine if I could clear out all the toxins I'm carryin'*, he thought excitedly.

"I'd love to try my parents again, if that's okay?"

"Good idea, go for it," Sam replied, folding up the big map on the floor. It was now dark outside and Denise was already in the kitchen with Bob, preparing the dinner juice.

Dave found himself back in the big, comfy office chair dialing home. This time his Mum answered and was very happy to hear his voice.

"Are you okay Dave? We've been really worried about you!"

"Yeah Mum… I'm all good. Actually feelin' better than I have for months. Bob brought me down to his brother's Eco Retreat and I don't think I've ever rested so much in my whole life. It's been amazing."

"Oh… that's good. We knew you'd be okay, but after ten days it is nice to hear from you."

"Yeah, I'm sorry. The time's just flown past, and I knew Bob had already filled you in. Oh, thanks for throwin' some money in for fuel as well. That was a real surprise."

"That's fine. You know we love to help out. Bob seems like a nice enough guy and I know you get along well with him. Your father's not so sure though. Reckons he looks like the original surfie bum and doesn't trust him at all. He'd kill me if he knew I gave him $100."

"It's true. He does appear a bit wild, but he's really lookin' after me and I'm learnin' lots."

"Oh, that's good… Listen, your father's here. He'd love to speak with you. I'll put him on." There was some fumbling around on the other end and unexpectedly Dave began feeling nervous.

"G'day Dave, how's it all going?"

"Yeah, really goin' good. Just stayin' down at Bob's brother's place. It's in the bush, about half hour out of Ulludulla. I've even got my own cabin. Been helpin' out around the place each day and they're really nice people. I'm startin' to feel heaps better too."

"That's great. Good spot that Ulludulla. Had some good fishin' there years ago. Remember getting those prawns with your brother that night, when you were kids."

"Yeah… I'd forgotten about that."

The tone in his dad's voice changed: "So when are you coming back for work? They called yesterday to see where you were. You'll lose that job if you're not careful!" came his stern words, thumping through the phone line.

Dave was torn. He needed the dollars, but the idea of loosing his job actually felt like a relief. "Yeah... I dunno," Dave said, beginning to crumble. "I'm thinkin' I might go west with Bob."

His dad fired back: "What are you gunna do for work? You've got a solid job here y'know. They've been good to you these people. You don't want to go stuffin' them around!"

"Look Dad, just relax. I'm workin' it out."

"Don't tell me to relax. I didn't bring you up to go gallivanting around the country with some stinking-bloody-hippie. You've got a lot to learn young man."

Dave could feel himself starting to see red and decided ending the call was the only option. He could've argued for hours, but knew this time 'round it was a total waste of energy. He took a deep breath. "Listen. Bob's a good bloke y'know. And if the hardware calls again, tell 'em I quit. The job sucks anyway. I've gotta go. See ya."

Dave quickly hung up the phone to escape the barrage of abuse, which he knew was just about to magnify ten fold. His dad was ferocious. *Fuck him, what does he know, angry old cunt!* Dave thought, shaking his head. Then it hit him... he'd just quit his job. It kinda came in the heat of the moment, but as it began to sink in, a feeling of immense freedom shot through him.

Dave sat there in the chair for a few minutes, integrating. His headache had completely gone. He was feeling super-energised and his body felt bigger than normal. There was so much happening inside him, he couldn't quite figure it out. What had become clear though, was going home to live with his family, returning to the city, or working at the hardware store again, was not going to happen. He now knew deep down, there was no going back.

After the dinner juice, Dave felt the need to have some time alone and went back to his cabin. His whole world was transforming before his eyes. He'd almost gone a whole day without food and also just realised his old life, as he knew it, was a thing of the past. There was no doubt that he would now join Bob and Freedom on the adventure. He didn't have a clue what he'd do for money but his body was buzzing with a new sense of independence. He lay in bed for an hour before drifting off to sleep, his mind alive with all the possibilities of what was to come.

The alarm clock rang louder than ever the next morning. Apart from the continuing cries of the rooster, it sounded very still outside and Dave awoke feeling clear and light. He went straight outside to the orange tree on auto-pilot and as his arm reached up to grab one, he remembered he had another day to endure on the juice fast. He was full-power hungry this morning. Standing there at the tree, he felt to not eat for another whole day would be impossible!

The best distraction he could think of was to get away from the tree as soon as possible and go for a walk to his sunrise rock. The weather had totally cleared and it was a magical morning. There was an extra chill in the air and Dave grabbed a thick jacket for the walk. It seemed a lot further than usual and his legs were weak. All he could think of was food. Finally, he arrived at the rock, sitting down exhausted. A whole day and night had passed and all he'd lived on was juice and water. Considering the circumstances, he wasn't feeling too bad at all. A little light-headed and wobbly, but in general he was fine. The sun was already up and there wasn't a breath of wind. Everything was quiet... quieter than usual.

The last day on the juice was a real challenge. During the afternoon the metallic taste and headache came back. He was ready for it this time though and didn't give it too much energy. They all spent the day in the garden, planting and doing fun things to keep the time passing. To help with the food cravings, a morning tea and afternoon juice was also created.

Dave slept early again that night and to his surprise, he slept really well. He woke before the rooster even crowed and was out at the orange tree eating as it let the first cry of the morning go. He was ravenous, and delighted in devouring three juicy big ones, like a starved, wild animal. Just to have something to chew again was awesome. Breakfast could not come soon enough. He imagined the table set out with oats, toast, nuts and all the other goodies.

Today, he didn't quite have the energy for a walk, so he just took an early morning tour of the fruit trees and veggie gardens, sampling the produce as he went. It was another chilly morning. He felt proud and almost as if he was walking through his own garden.

It was inspiring. The whole place looked incredible.

Breakfast was earlier than usual and he thoroughly enjoyed every mouthful. The taste of the food was enhanced and his appreciation had gone to a new level. *How could healthy food taste this good?* he thought, lathering some coconut oil onto his toast. It was a real celebration breakfast. The vibration was high and everyone had an extra sparkle in their eyes. And as usual, there was no shortage of laughter.

It was decided they would head off in two days time. On one hand, Dave felt like he could've stayed there forever and on the other, he realised it was finally time to move on. He had no real idea of what lay ahead but from what Bob had shared, the adventure was only just beginning.

The next couple of days were spent preparing for the journey. Dave helped Bob do a basic service on the van and it was cleaned and stocked with supplies. They loaded up a big cardboard box full of fruit and stacked the little fridge with veggies. Bob even burned some herbs and fanned the smoke throughout the van. It actually smelt a bit like pot. Dave was sure he wasn't a stoner and decided not to ask any questions. It was weird though, especially when Bob started mumbling prayers for a safe journey on the road ahead.

The day to leave arrived. It was grey and overcast with light drizzle. The mood at breakfast was heavier than usual, as everyone (especially the kids) realised the extended family would be breaking up. Sam managed to lighten the vibe by putting on some funky tunes after breakfast and sharing with Bob and Dave just how grateful he was for their help since they'd been there. And the gratitude went both ways with Bob and Dave thanking the family over and over again.

Denise gifted Dave with a writing book and suggested to him it would be helpful to start writing a diary or jotting down his ideas. He gave her a big hug.

"You've all been so good to me. I appreciate it a lot," Dave said.

"You are very welcome," Denise responded. "We've loved having you here and you're welcome any time."

After a bunch more goodbyes and hugs, the final bits and pieces went into the van and they were on their way.

8. CRAZY CHARLEY

Dave leaned out the window of the old Kombi, taking one last look at the property and waving back to the family. He wound the window up and rubbed his hands together quickly.

"Thanks so much for takin' me to your bro's place. I'm feelin' heaps better. It's almost been like a dream," he said gratefully.

"Sweet. Yeah man, you even look different to what you did a few weeks back. It's like your eyes are bigger or somethin'. You've got more of a glow goin' on!"

Freedom rattled away up the tree lined road. The windscreen wipers screeched across the glass with each stroke. Bob turned the music up to drown out the sound and then flowed into some of his groovy, driving dance moves, which got the passenger smiling. Bob was always having so much fun. He was like a child in a man's body. The way he laughed, danced and could constantly see the bright side of life, was inspiring. Dave loved hanging out with him. It was a real breath of fresh air. The idea that all adults had to be serious was fading from his brain rapidly.

"Ever driven a Kombi before dude? We've got a bunch of drivin' to do and I reckon it'll be cool if we share the load."

"Nah, I haven't... but I'm willin' to give it a shot." Dave replied.

"Awesome, it's easy! I reckon you're ready to take your relationship with Freedom to the next level. I'm pretty good for the next couple of hours man, but if we can take shifts after that I'd be stoked. That way, we'll be there before we know it!"

A whole new adventure lay ahead and it was great to be on the road again. Rather than following the coast, they decided to cut inland over the mountains to save time and money. If they drove all day, every day, it would take them a week to get to their destination. Bob had done the trip plenty of times and was in no real hurry. His view was that if it took a couple of weeks, that was fine. The most important thing was that they were having fun and with the space the two of them were in, it was guaranteed.

The next few days were all pretty much the same. Driving, driving and more driving. Going up over the mountains was freezing and Freedoms little old heater barely cut the mustard. At one stage, Bob was driving with his sleeping bag wrapped around him which was a sight to see. It was such a practical vehicle to travel in. Everything was available right at your fingertips.

Dave slowly got a handle on driving the old bus and after a few days behind the wheel, he had it mastered. After hours and hours of sitting, with numb bums and stiff backs, they were realising the importance of moving the body. Every so often Bob would pull over for a piss and one of his famous dance breaks. He'd pull off the road in some random location – generally where there wasn't another soul in sight – pump up the stereo and then just go wild. It was bananas! A thirty-something year old man, with hair, beard, arms and legs going everywhere. The first few times it happened, Dave was in shock. He became certain that his travelling buddy was bonkers. He couldn't work out whether to laugh or run away.

After Bob's constant invitation to join in, he eventually couldn't resist. And besides, there was nowhere to run anyway. By the third official dance break, something inside of him let go and Dave joined the madman. He fully made sure there was no possibility of onlookers and then gingerly started shaking his body. Half way through the song, he realised the fun potential available and something in him came alive. The African drums pumping out of the van worked their wonders, and all the judgements and fears he'd been harbouring, simply fell away.

Bob was astounded... Firstly to see Dave's liberation, and secondly, he now had himself a dancing partner! Once they'd had enough, the two of them stood there in the sunshine, laughing at the whole situation and celebrating Dave's new-found freedom. It was the first time he'd ever danced without the help of alcohol, and he enjoyed every minute of it!

It had been three long days on the road and a hot shower was calling. Dave was still in the same clothes he'd had on since they'd left Sam's place and there was definitely a bit of stink going on. Especially now that he was taking part in the sweaty dance breaks... they'd just topped things off! In a few more hours they'd reach a town with a caravan park, where Bob had previously paid a couple of bucks for a shower. Apparently the manager there was a real character and Bob was hoping he'd be around.

His wish came true and an interesting night unfolded. Charley was the manager's name and even though Bob had only been there briefly two or three times before, Charley remembered him. The caravan park was almost empty and when they pulled in, Charley came shooting out from reception to greet them. He was an overweight man around the age of fifty, with a big red nose and chubby cheeks. He reminded Dave of Santa Claus, but a shorts wearing Aussie version.

"Hi Bob, welcome back! I was wondering when you and the old van would be coming through again. You after your yearly shower, hey?" he said, before exploding into laughter, exactly like Santa Claus and not stopping for over thirty seconds. Charley's laugh was outrageous. Dave couldn't believe his ears. It was a proper, full-belly 'Ho! Ho! Ho!' that was louder than the engine of the Kombi and finished with a rough, wheezing sound, like he was choking on something or about to have a heart attack.

Before Bob even had a chance to say hello and introduce Dave, they'd already been invited for dinner and there was no way in the world Santa Claus was accepting a 'no'. This guy was out of control!

"Park your bongo van over there and I'll get the shower key!" Charley barked, still chuckling and wheezing at his joke.

The hot shower was well received and complemented with some warm, clean clothes, left Dave feeling like a new man.

Charley's house and the reception area to the park, were all one building. There was no one around at the front desk so Bob rang the bell. "Are you there Charley?"

"Is that you, ya freeloaders?" came a voice from the next room, followed by raucous laughter. *This is going to be an interesting night*, Dave thought, not knowing quite how to take this new friend. Charley entered the room with a large beer bottle in one hand and a devilish grin.

"From compost to rose petals hey! Is that perfume you've got on Bob?" he asked, accompanied by more noise. "Come on through and meet the gang."

They followed Charley down a dark hallway and went through a door, into what looked to be the living area. Far out! It looked like a bomb had gone off in there. The place was a mess. There were dirty plates and glasses stacked up on the table, dozens of empty beer bottles and even a big-old-black-dog, asleep on the couch. Dave could hear kids in another room and some noise at the far end of the living area, he guessed to be the kitchen. *And he was complaining about our smell!* Dave thought to himself.

Charley kicked a few things aside to clear a path. "Come and meet the boss," he said, walking towards the kitchen, followed closely by the two guests, looking around in disbelief. The kitchen revealed even more mess and a short, thin, vacant-looking, dark haired woman. "Sweetheart, this is Bob and…? What's your name young fella? I haven't even been introduced. Old slack ass here," he said, pointing to Bob, "is a little slow on the introductions!"

Dave put out his hand for a shake, realising this would not be a hugging sort of situation. "I'm Dave," he said, in a guarded manner.

"Well Dave and Bob, this is my other half Sharon and I don't want either of you getting any ideas!" Charley said, followed by his loud and now extremely annoying laughter. Sharon immediately shrank away, back into the sink where she was doing the dishes, embarrassed and obviously feeling very uncomfortable. Charley's laughter subsided and there was a moment of awkward silence. He took a big gulp of his beer and the show continued: "How's the pizza's lookin' sweetheart? I could eat a horse and chase the jockey!" he bellowed.

"It'll be ready in five minutes," his wife replied, in

a high pitched, squeaky voice.

Dave felt like he'd been transported into some other world. How could people live like this? Why would they even choose to? After his heart-warming time at Sam's place, this was definitely a taste of the other end of the scale. It was actually really sad. Bob was very quiet and Dave guessed he was feeling the same way.

The pizza was served up onto a corner of the table that had the least amount of junk on it. Some of the other mess was cleared away and paper towels were passed around for plates. The kids were playing computer games in their bedroom and after half a dozen stern demands from Charley, they eventually appeared. Two girls, about thirteen and fifteen and a younger brother of probably eight or nine. They were all pale-looking, overweight and didn't say much at all. When Dave said hello they all just nodded their heads, mumbled a bit and didn't even look at him. Who knows if they were shy or just not used to visitors. But hey, this was a caravan park! He had a truck load of questions but not a lot of answers.

The pizzas were from the supermarket freezer, with the fake looking cheese, slightly overcooked and very crunchy. Dave used to eat these babies all the time but after a couple of pieces, his stomach was saying, please no more. He was eating more out of politeness than anything. Bob had barely touched his. The kids grabbed their share and retreated back to the bedroom.

The next half hour rocked and rolled between

Charley's wild jokes, his laughter and a thick, awkward silence. The dinner guests sat there flabbergasted, watching the whole scenario unfold. It was getting to the point where they both needed to get out of there as quickly as possible... The fun was long gone. Charley was getting drunker and his jokes had gone from fairly light to plain old nasty.

Suddenly Bob stood up, firmly announcing: "Well, thank you both. It's been a big day and now it's time for us to call it a night!" There was a clarity and sharpness in his voice that Dave had rarely heard. It reminded him of the morning he'd come tapping on his window. It was the sort of voice that no one can argue with and there was an unmistakable strength about it, which caught Charley absolutely off guard. Bob laid a $5 note on the table, stating clearly it was for the showers and began heading for the exit door, followed closely by Dave.

Charley didn't know what to do and sat there looking puzzled. The stinking hippie from the blue van had revealed a new side of himself. All he could muster as they walked away was: "Okay... we'll see you tomorrow then," and for once, silence followed instead of laughter. The two escapees hurried down the dark hallway, out the door and headed straight for Freedom waiting patiently in the car park for them.

"Jump in, let's get the hell outta here!" Bob said, firing up the engine.

It was still only early evening and even though they didn't like driving at night due to trucks and kangaroos, tonight was a unique exception. There was no way they were going to spend another minute there. Dave was relieved to be back in the van and on the road again. The whole vibe of Charley's house and pizza evening was dark, dirty and depressing. Charley was a crazy man and very challenging to be around. For the next hour they took it slowly and spent the time debriefing about what'd just happened.

A lot of interesting topics were covered. Such as alcohol and drug abuse and how it can tear families apart. The challenges of relationships and some of the pitfalls of the computer age. They could see the stark difference between Sam and Denise's children and the kids they'd just encountered. Even though they were younger, the confidence, aliveness and joy that was oozing from Jarrah and Sandy was obviously due to their environment. In comparison, these kids they'd just met were like dead robots. It was sad to see but unfortunately so common.

Dave saw the similarities in many of his friends and their brothers and sisters. It wasn't just the kids either. Bob shared his insight that it was a disease of the modern age:

"We sit in our cars on the way to work, sit in front of our computers all day long, then go home, where we sit down and watch TV or spend more time on the computer... it's just nuts!"

"Yeah, ya not wrong there. Guess I was pretty lucky to be so into sport and surfin'. Played the odd computer game, but was never really into it."

They were both getting tired. It had been another big day behind the wheel. Bob turned off the highway and eventually found a safe place to sleep for the night in amongst some trees. The roof of the van was popped up and Dave began preparing his bed. He'd been given the 'upstairs bed' while Bob folded the couch down and organised his space in a very familiar way. Dave loved being up in the top section. It was like his own, private little room and he slept well up there. To be able to just pull up anytime, anywhere and have a sound night's sleep was a bonus.

The next morning was cold and to get the blood pumping, Bob inspired Dave to go for a jog with him. They were out in the middle of nowhere surrounded by low scrub and the odd pocket of trees. The air was fresh and there wasn't another soul around for miles. What a great way to start the day. Once back at the van, a quality stretching session went down. Luckily, Bob had two yoga mats on hand and schooled Dave in on some basic yoga postures.

He explained how he'd discovered yoga in California when he was about Dave's age and it had transformed his life. He revealed that the morning after his very first class, he'd literally sprung out of bed, feeling more balanced and alive than ever before. He vividly remembered going surfing that day and was so 'in tune', he couldn't fall off if he tried. This was a good sell and Dave was suddenly extra interested. He'd done plenty of stretching in his time but nothing like the moves Bob was showing him. To stretch out, after days on end in the car left their bodies liberated and alive. Dave especially enjoyed the relaxation at the end of the session and almost drifted off to sleep. After a healthy breakfast in the warm morning sun, they were on the road again.

Ahead of them was another full day behind the wheel. The morning fitness routine had left them both feeling pumped. Every time they stopped for fuel, the skipping rope came out and they took it in turns bouncing away to the delight of onlookers. Both of them were keen to become fit and strong for the upcoming surf adventures and it was happening. Dave's energy had almost totally balanced out and he was feeling awesome!

Bob explained his idea that there is unlimited energy available to us all, every moment of every day, and a big part of human suffering and fatigue is when we close off to that energy.

"It's so important to keep the energy moving through us," he reasoned. "That's why I love dancing, running, surfing and yoga, 'cause once that energy is moving freely through me, I feel fantastic!" Bob reached across and pointed to a small, square, brightly-coloured sticker on the dashboard which read, MOVE IT OR LOSE IT! and then had a good laugh.

Hour after hour behind the wheel unfolded. They were passing through a spectacular part of the country and it blew Dave's mind. The road was dead straight for hundreds of kilometres. It was flat and barren, with small salt bushes scattered here and there. Such an ancient landscape. They passed the odd car but apart from that, it was just wide, open space for miles around.

Bob had a whopping CD collection which included

inspirational talks from a variety of people about life, with tips on how to approach the usual day-to-day challenges differently. Dave had no idea that these sorts of things were available and he was beginning to understand why the lanky Californian was such a positive man. By listening to this sort of wisdom, it could truly change the way you see the world. Even after a few hours, Dave had a renewed sense of positivity and appreciation for life. It was like magic!

Two more long days behind the wheel followed before they arrived at a small, coastal township that was well known for its big wave surfing. It was official... they were now on the other side of the country! Bob had spent time here over the years and had experienced some very memorable surf sessions.

The day was drawing to a close and they made for the local big wave spot to check it out before dark. As they pulled into the car park, Dave was gob-smacked with what lay before him. He'd never seen waves of that size... anywhere. This place was surely living up to its reputation. Dave had seen loads of Hawaiian surf movies over the years and that's exactly what it looked like. Only it was real, right there in front of him... It was as if the whole ocean was moving.

The car park overlooked the reef and the entire bay. It was spectacular! Bob explained the set-up and where you would normally surf. It was hard to make it all out though, as it looked like a giant washing machine. They both jumped out to stretch their legs and firmly plant their feet on the ground. They'd made it successfully from one side of the country to the other and a few celebration high fives were thrown around.

The sun was sinking into the ocean which just added to the scene. It seemed a lot of the locals came there to watch the sunset and check the surf. There were loads of cars and people everywhere. Bob got talking with a tall, strong looking character who let on that the following morning was going to be all-time. An offshore wind was forecast and it was predicted that the swell would hang in there.

9. FREEING THE LION

Dave woke early to the thunderous roar of Mother Ocean. He'd tossed and turned all night with a stiff wind rattling the canvas walls of his little room, combined with the relentless pounding of the waves. Unzipping the corner of his window, he got a glimpse of what he could hear. Overnight, the ocean had transformed itself into clean lines of swell, stacked all the way to the horizon. The stiff offshore wind had done more than just rattle his bedroom! There were already half a dozen cars in the car park and a few guys with wetsuits on, waxing their boards.

They must be super keen, Dave thought, as it was freezing outside.

"How's it lookin'?" came a sleepy voice from the lower storey.

"Sooooo clean and sooooo BIG!" came the report from above.

"Oh yeah! Man, I'm out there." Bob instantly pulled himself out of his cosy bed and put his big jacket on in preparation for the morning chill. The sun wasn't up yet and the sky was a combination of blue, grey and purple. Dave stayed rugged up in bed, studying the waves through the fly-screen mesh. He could see now exactly what Bob had been talking about last night. The washing machine had been replaced by a huge, grinding left hander. There were already three surfers out there and a couple more paddling out. It was looking very Hawaiian again and Dave was still yet to see anyone catch a wave. There was a real buzz in the air and a few more guys ran past the van, talking excitedly amongst themselves. Under their arms they carried extra long big wave boards and looked ready for action.

These were serious waves. Even to get out to the take-off spot was a two hundred metre paddle. And the offshore breeze was so powerful that it wasn't allowing the surfers to actually paddle into the waves. Eventually, someone on a red board caught a beast and rode it successfully into the channel, to the delight of those watching from the car park, who responded with hoots and beeping horns. Bob was pumped to get amongst it and already had his wetsuit on.

"Are you comin' out Dave?" he asked, with uncertainty.

"No way... It's monstrous out there. Plus I've only got my short board. I wouldn't even be able to get near those things."

Bob slid the larger of his two boards from the van and began to wax up.

"That wind should drop out in the next few hours which'll make it loads easier. But I can't hang here just watchin', I love this wave way too much. If you get frothed you know where I'll be!" Bob threw the wax back in, slid the door shut, took off across the grass and down the stairs. Dave was torn. He really wanted to join Bob and at the same time didn't have the equipment. The wipeout he'd had recently was playing on his mind as well and today was two or three times as big as that... Easily! His energy was back and he was feeling very alive though. Part of him knew he'd be okay out there and at the same time he was nervous and afraid. He was in a strange space... his mind going crazy. He was even angry at himself for not going surfing.

There were a few oranges left in the box and Dave climbed down out of bed, rugged up, grabbed one and went outside for his new morning ritual. Starting the day with a piece of fresh fruit felt so natural to him. As soon as he was outside with the cool wind and a mouthful of orange, he felt much better. He reflected back to the previous day and one of the inspirational CD's Bob was playing. The lady had suggested that whenever you're not feeling so good, to just stop and think of five things you are grateful for in your life at that moment. Apparently it was a way to change your vibration. Dave liked the simplicity of it and decided to give it a shot.

Okay, number one, he thought, taking another mouthful of orange. *I am grateful for this delicious, juicy orange... that was an easy one! Number two...* He stopped, looked around and realised that he was standing on the grass, overlooking the biggest, best waves he'd ever seen in real life. Out to the east the sun was rising from behind the hill, throwing luminous, soft colours across the sky.

I am grateful to be here this morning, in this epic spot! Wow, he was feeling better already. This was becoming fun. He walked over to the stairs and down onto the beach. *Number three...I am grateful for my energy coming back and the fact I'm feeling healthier and healthier every day!* Dave was on a roll now. *Number four... I am grateful for the opportunity to step out of my old life and start an awesome, new adventure!*

It was much nicer down on the beach due to the protection from the cool, offshore breeze. Dave could see the spot from where you paddle out and the waves looked even better from this vantage point. Someone dropped into a monster and he could tell from the ultra-casual style that it was Bob. Instantly, number five popped straight into his head. *I'm so grateful for havin' Bob as my friend. It's as if he's saved my life!*

Dave watched closely as Bob rode his wave till the end and stood tall as he pulled off, throwing his arms high into the air. It was all-time Bob-style and a pleasure to watch. The gratitude process had worked and Dave now felt much lighter and appreciative of his whole life. The confusion, fear and anger had totally disappeared.

"Holy shit... that stuff actually works!" he said out loud, followed by a little chuckle of disbelief. He took a walk to explore the beach, rocks and the entire bay. It was a magical place and apart from the surfers and the car park, there was no one around. He discovered a beautiful secluded beach and a river. The whole place was so different from the east coast. It was raw, wild and seemingly untouched. The huge, pounding waves were awe-inspiring. The power and the energy of this ocean left Dave feeling strong, alive and very much at home.

By the time he got back to the van, the sun was fully up and Bob was already out of the water. He reckoned it was still way too windy out there which was making things hard, especially with the size of the waves. That was a good surprise to Dave's ears and helped melt away any no-surf stress he was still carrying.

The usual breakfast of Bob's famous muesli, combined with all the extras was rustled together.

"Man... what a day!" Bob expressed wholeheartedly, with a mouthful of muesli. "This place is just oozing the Aloha spirit." He continued, putting on his best Californian surf movie commentary voice: "While Dave and Bob sat in the car park that fine autumn morning, blown about by the cool offshore breeze, they could hardly believe their eyes. The sparkling Indian Ocean continued to neatly stack corduroy swell lines all the way to the horizon. The day that was unfolding before them would go down in the history books of surfing forever!" Both of them broke into laughter and Dave half choked on his breakfast.

"Is that you Bob?" came an excited voice from the other side of the car park. They both turned to see who it was.

"Hey Geoff," Bob replied enthusiastically, getting up to reunite with his old friend and share a big hug. "Man, its been almost a year hey."

"That's true. So good to see you. Wasn't sure if you'd be comin' over this year. You goin' north again?"

"For sure man... got an apprentice with me this year too!" he said, with a laugh. "Geoff, this is Dave."

Geoff walked over to Dave with a big smile and shook his hand. "Pleased to meet you mate. You must've done somethin' right, hangin' out with this character!" he said, gesturing back at Bob.

Dave nodded in agreement. "Yeah... I'm pretty stoked hey."

Bob made Geoff up a bowl of muesli to join the 'breakfast club', with the best view ever. For the next half hour, the stories and jokes they shared were mind boggling. The two of them were like long, lost brothers and Dave just sat back enjoying every minute of the show. Geoff had his car loaded with big wave boards and offered up an old 7'6" for Dave to use. It had been snapped and fixed but it would be far better than his little 6'2" beach-break board. What an offer! It was too good to refuse and he jumped at it.

The wind was starting to die out and the swell had dropped a little. The sun was shining and there were still only a handful of surfers tackling the swells. The two older legends schooled Dave as best they could about the ins and outs of surfing the place. Where to paddle out, which waves to look for and which ones to avoid, where to swim if you lost your board and that was just the beginning! It was a lot of information to take in but it was clear and all made sense. Dave was energised, excited and in good hands.

He had never even carried a board of this size before, let alone surfed one. He'd ridden a few Malibus but they were nothing like this. They all paddled out together, staying in a close pack and continuing Dave's education. The water was clean, clear and refreshing. As they approached the take-off zone, a set of five or six large waves moved in, thundering onto the reef. The first two were ridden, while the other surfers scrambled to avoid the rest of the set landing fair on them. From the water these waves looked twice as big as they did from the car park. Dave lay there on his board totally spellbound by what he'd just witnessed. Mother Ocean at her most spectacular! These weren't actually waves, they were moving mountains of water and so big, that it looked like they were breaking slowly as they moved in over the reef.

Bob and Geoff kept paddling feverishly over to where the waves were breaking, while Dave intelligently decided to sit in the channel for a while, to get a handle on what was happening. You could tell Geoff was a local 'cause he was so at home out there. He was catching wave after wave and having loads of fun. Even after nasty wipeouts he'd come up laughing and go back out for more. Bob was more reserved and always made sure he was in the right spot at the right time. He caught two huge waves from way out the back. After each wave, he paddled over to Dave to see how he was going.

Half an hour passed and Dave was ready to move in closer to the peak, to better his chances of catching one. He paddled over cautiously with Geoff just after a big set had gone through.

"Righto Dave, we've got about ten minutes before the next set. We'll see if we can get you into one of these in-betweeners!"

"Sounds good," the attentive student replied.

"Okay, this one over the back. Paddle this way," Geoff said, precisely and quickly. Dave followed Geoff and got sight of his wave. If this was an in-betweener, he wasn't going anywhere near one of the sets! Adrenalin coursed through his body but he was unusually calm at the same time. "Righto, you're in the spot… It's all yours. Go. Go. Go!"

Dave sat up on his board and swung it around. He knew if he wasn't fast enough he'd have a repeat of his last reef experience, so he dug deep and paddled his guts out. He was in the perfect spot and the wave picked him up early.

"Go. Go. Gooooo… Yooooohhhhhh!!" was all he could hear as he jumped to his feet. It felt like he was standing on the roof of a two-storey house or about to ski down a steep mountain. It was too much for his mind, which thankfully shut off. Dave's years of surfing experience kicked in as he slid down the face at high speed... focused, alert and ready for anything.

With that same tenacity and focus he leaned into a big bottom turn and went flying down the line, out-running the wave and making it safely to the channel. He threw his arms into the air and gave a massive hoot which was echoed by Geoff, back out in the take-off area. His mind was gone. He just sat there on his board for a few moments in wonder, with a huge smile on his face. He'd done it! He'd conquered a big reef break wave! Any fear that he had left in him was transformed and all that remained was excitement. He was ready for more. Paddling back out he saw both Geoff and Bob catch spectacular waves and hooted like a wild man from the channel.

He paddled straight out to where the other surfers had positioned themselves, awaiting their next ride. The wind had all but died right out and only a light offshore remained. The mid-morning sun had some relieving warmth in it and the ocean was a deep, emerald green. The adrenalin continued to pump strongly through his body.

"I heard you got a beauty!" exclaimed Bob, paddling up beside him, giving him a massive high five. He was so happy for Dave and amazed that he'd even gathered the courage to surf these waves. It was after all, a serious day.

"Out the back!" came a short, sharp burst from Geoff as he quickly stroked past them both, his eyes fixed on the horizon. Dave had been lost in the story of his wave and hadn't even seen the approaching set. The scramble was on.

"Dave... paddle this way!" Bob suggested, as he made for the channel. The instructions were of no use at this point. Dave's world now revolved around the mountain of water he was faced with. It was like an apartment block moving through the ocean, about to fall over right in front of him. No matter what he did, at this point he was in trouble. He was trying to flee but it was all too late. There was no possible way he could fight... So the last of his survival instincts kicked in. He froze.

Bob saw what was happening and commanded him in a loud, sharp voice: "Throw your board Dave, THROW your board!" This snapped Dave out of it. He looked across at Bob who was only ten metres away, also in the same predicament. Dave took a deep breath, slid off the side of his board and started swimming for the bottom as if a shark was chasing him.

KAABOOOOOOOOM!!! The wave landed right on top of him detonating like an atom bomb. He was overcome instantly by the turbulence and this time the washing machine was set on super-maxi cycle. The legrope almost yanked his left limb clean off, before the tension completely disappeared. All he could do was surrender and go with it, as Geoff had suggested in his pre-surf schooling. It was far too powerful to even consider struggling to get back to the top. Eventually he surfaced, gasping for air, his board nowhere to be seen. Bob was still close by him and looked very happy to see him emerge.

Luckily they'd both been washed into deeper

water and the next wave that hit them was nothing compared to the first. After swimming under a few more and finally getting their breath back, Bob paddled over to Dave and managed to get him on the front of his board. Dave's legs were spread out and his ass was jammed right in Bob's face. It was an awkward way to rescue his young mate, but they eventually managed to get their balance and make some ground. The duo was blown apart a couple of times by some ferocious white water and finally reached a calmer area, closer to shore, where Dave's board was bobbing around. Luckily it had somehow managed to avoid getting smashed onto the rocks.

"Thanks Bob... that's one I owe ya," Dave gasped.

"All good bro. You weren't the only one freakin' out then. That was heavy!"

They called it a day on the surf front and were both happy to have their feet back on the sand. Even though Dave had almost drowned once again surfing a reef break, something had changed. By heeding Geoff's advice, he hadn't panicked as much this time and handled the intensity of the situation quite well. The key seemed to be all about relaxing and saving your energy, which can be a challenge when you're stuck under Niagara Falls! Dave was still pumped about the wave he'd successfully ridden and it made him feel twenty feet tall. The fact he'd paddled out and faced one of his biggest fears was extremely liberating. He felt strong, alive and as though he could do anything.

The rest of the morning was spent recapping the surf, eating and enjoying the whole scene. The waves continued to roll in and from all reports, it had been the best day in a long while. All the locals were friendly and the vibration was high. Dave lay down on the grass in the midday sun and melted into the ground, his new-found freedom and ease continuing to sprout in his body. Just to have the time and space to lie down and not be anyone, or do anything or have to go anywhere... What a life!

They decided to head back into town to fuel up and get a few needed supplies. The petrol kitty had run dry again and Dave only had $300 left to his name. He assumed his usual role at the service station and as he cleaned the windscreen of the van, he questioned himself as to how it would be possible to make some more dollars. Rather than freaking out about not having enough money, he decided to focus on what he could do to obtain some more. Bob's inspiring CD's had been having more effect than he realised.

They both put another $50 each into the old sock and Dave's heart skipped a beat, realising that his $300 had now become $250. Bob went in to pay and took forever, eventually returning with some local news.

"Apparently there's some market on today at the top of town. It's one of the biggest of the year. There will be hundreds of people there and I'm amped to check it out!"

"I'm keen as. Let's do it!" Dave replied, with a sparkle in his eye.

On the way there, Bob shared some stories of his younger days travelling and busking at markets to earn some extra dollars. Dave loved his yarns and then the penny dropped.

"You know what? Your busking career has just started again and I'm your new sidekick!" he said, with great enthusiasm. Bob laughed loudly and then cottoned onto the idea. He had his favourite drum tucked away in the van with a bunch of other percussion instruments and happily agreed to join in on Dave's grand plan.

"The funds are almost gone so I figured I'd better start gettin' creative," Dave said. "Those CD's we've been listenin' to have really inspired me and after this mornin's surf, I'm feelin' invincible!" He was beginning to come alive more than ever and Bob was really enjoying the transformation. He always knew Dave's potential but to actually see it unfolding before his eyes, made his heart sing.

"Here we are man. The Margaret River Show!" Bob sang out, as they strolled up to the gate. The market was buzzing alright. The colours, stalls, variety of food vendors… they even had rides and a jumping castle for the kids. There was no mucking around. Bob called on his seasoned market knowledge and with drum-in-hand marched straight to the busiest part of the market. Dave followed closely behind sporting a tambourine, tapping sticks and this funny little egg shaker with a smiley face on it.

They set up under a tree just off to the side of the

food area, where over a hundred people were gathered having their lunch. It was a festive scene and if they were going to make any money, this was the place. Bob prepared his hat by emptying his wallet into it with a handful of coins and even threw in a five and ten dollar note. Turning to Dave, he said quietly:

"This just gets 'em thinkin' man... if everyone else is throwin' in the big bucks, we better as well. It's an old buskers trick."

To Bob's surprise, Dave jumped up and at the top of his voice, began: "Ladies and Gentlemen. Thank you for coming down today! Please put your hands together for Bob on the drum! All the way from Ca-li-for-ni-AAAA... Take it away Bob!!"

Holey moley. He sat back down absolutely astonished. He hadn't done anything out of the blue like that for ages, and it felt amazing. His voice was LOUD! He'd not only shocked himself but the onlookers as well. They all looked up from their lunches to see what the fuss was about.

Bob began and was holding a good rhythm on the drum. He could really play and it sounded awesome. Dave stood up, grabbed hold of the tambourine and acted like he knew exactly what he was doing. His marketing technique had worked and a few people started gathering around and moving to the beats. Soon there were kids everywhere, dancing, playing around and having a ball. The adults were grooving away behind them and a little concert was unfolding. To make things even better, money was flowing quickly into the hat.

Dave kept rattling away on the tambourine in time and even began dancing himself. He could not believe what was happening, right in front of his eyes. Bob was also starting to get right into it and even began singing like a Native American chief. The crowd was impressed and the hat continued filling up. After half an hour, the energy had died away and both Bob and Dave were exhausted. What a day it had been... Full power! The drum stopped and the crowd slowly eased away.

"Thank you for your generosity ladies and gentlemen. We hope you've enjoyed the show!" Dave bellowed, finalising his short speech with a shaking tambourine. They looked at each other and then down at the hat, which was overflowing with coins and notes. Their eyes connected again and they both burst out laughing.

"In all my years on the busk, I've never had such overwhelmingly quick success. Thanks to you, my new marketin' manager." Bob said, laughing again. "Okay Dave, let's get the hell out of here before anyone wants a cut of our takin's!"

They ran like kids being chased, back to Freedom to tally their dollars. Excitement and joy pulsed through their bodies. Dave counted the coins while Bob sorted through the notes. In total, they'd made $237. It was incredible.

"I didn't even know that much could fit into my hat!" Bob laughed, shaking his head, astounded.

10. WELCOME TO PARADISE

The wind howled again all night and they awoke to some of the heaviest rain in history. Dave's bedroom had even sprung a leak! It possibly had something to do with it being so windy that the rain was actually going sideways. It was a miracle the van hadn't been blown over.

"Up anchor... we're going north!" were Bob's first words for the day, in his best pirate-voice, said with plenty of gusto to be heard above the storm outside.

"Aye-aye captain. I'll lower the hatch immediately!" rang out from the top deck.

Within minutes they were away. The road north was covered in branches, leaves and even the odd tree had fallen down in some places. Bob took it easy and skilfully negotiated Freedom through the obstacle course. What a ferocious night it'd been. Spirits were still high after yesterday's events and Dave could not stop talking about the wave he'd caught. He was still feeling twenty feet tall.

He was also completely rapt at how easily they'd made $237! Throughout his whole life, he'd believed that money doesn't come easily, or it doesn't grow on trees. Yesterday had blown those old theories out of the water.

"I still can't grasp just how easily we made all that money yesterday," he shared, looking across at Bob who was intently focused on the road.

"Wild huh... and that's the direction we're headin' my man! It's not just happenin' for us either, it's affectin' everyone across the planet. We're movin' away from a life of struggle and sacrifice to one of creativity and joy. It's really time for a change!" Bob exclaimed.

Dave knew exactly what he was talking about. "It seems my oldie's generation and many people still now, struggle and stress a lot about work and money. I know I certainly have. I'm gettin' the bigger picture now though. Imagine making loads of dollars and having fun at the same time!"

For the next few hours, his mind was alive with ideas of what else they could do. From surf tours, to selling fresh juice from the van and everything in-between... Even opening a Japanese restaurant! This kid was on fire. His creativity had been let loose and the long lost entrepreneur was waking up.

Finally they'd driven far enough north to escape the heavy rain. Breakfast was long overdue and Bob's ears were in need of a rest. Dave, with a mouthful of muesli, would be the perfect solution. In a day and a half, they'd arrive at the desert surf camp they had talked so much about. Here, Bob could truly school Dave in the art of reef break surfing and true, simple, healthy living. It would be the icing on the cake for his healing program.

The further north they drove, the better the weather became and it just kept getting warmer. After hundreds more kilometres, skipping and stretching at fuel stops, one unsuccessful busking performance outside a supermarket, and an endless, bumpy dirt road, they finally arrived at the Bluff. Bob was elated to be back.

"Welcome to Paradise!" he announced.

Dave was beside himself. After two days of non-stop talking, he was silent as they came up over the last hill revealing everything Bob had described. The place was truly captivating, like something out of a fantasy kid's book, crossed with a surf magazine. A long white beach stretched up into the corner, which turned into rugged, orange rocks and grassland. It was all set into a beautiful big bay, with inviting, crystal-clear blue water, shadowed by a towering mountain and headland. To top it all off there was a perfect, left hand point break, fanned by an offshore wind.

Dave remained silent, soaking it all up. Far out, there were even kangaroos on the headland! If paradise existed, then this was it! The old Kombi bounced down the last section of the corrugated road and pulled up in front of the booking office. Bob jumped out and Dave followed closely behind. A short, blonde-haired lady came out the door.

"Hey, aloha Bob... welcome back!" The two of them shared a hug.

"Great to see you Sally. It's so good to be back. I've brought a friend with me this year too," he gestured. "Sally, this is Dave, who lost his voice once we came over the hill." Sally approached Dave, putting out her hand:

"Well, you're definitely not the first one this place has left speechless, and I'm guessing you won't be the last." Sally had a strong, country-girl accent and looked right at home here in this desert paradise. They shook hands and Dave thought it'd be best if he came up with some words and proceeded to awkwardly let a few go:

"Happy to meet you," and then he warmed up a little. "What an amazing place you call home. It's sooo good here!"

The three of them walked back towards the office. "Come in guys," Sally said, holding the door open. It was a cosy little room with surfing pictures of the point hanging tastefully on the white walls. "You've virtually got the place to yourselves at the moment. There's only a dozen others here."

Bob looked excited and asked: "Are any of the shacks available?"

"There's two actually... the one in the valley and the love shack, closer to the point," Sally replied.

"We'll go the love shack for sure!" enthused Bob, totally surprised it was available, as it was one of the best in the camp ground.

"Rent's gone up a little this year guys. It's $10 each per night or $50 for the week."

"Too easy," Bob replied. "It's still one of the cheapest in the country."

Dave's entrepreneur side was still in top gear and he spoke up. "Hey Sally, I'm wonderin' if there's any jobs I can do around here to pay for my rent?"

"Definitely, Peter would love a hand with the rubbish run and the toilets if that interests you?"

"Yeah, for sure... I'm a rubbish and toilet specialist!" he added, with his new-found confidence. Dave was an ideas machine at the moment and there was an old looking massage table in the corner of the room that he'd noticed when they walked in. Already in his mind he was massaging tired surfers and whoever else to make a few extra dollars.

Imagine that, he thought. *My rent's already paid, and three or four good-value massages per week would cover the other costs.* He didn't know a heap about massage, but he'd received a few in his time from a friend of his mother's who was looking for guinea pigs during her training. With the way Dave was feeling at the moment, there was nothing he couldn't do!

"Sally, while I'm on a roll, I was wondering if that massage table over there is being used at the moment?"

"It's not ours mate. It belongs to Grace, a Dutch lady staying here. She does healing work and it's her spare one. If you want to use it, you'd best ask her. Her camp is a couple over from the love shack."

"Will do, thanks," he responded, feeling a little

deflated, thinking his idea might not be so good if he already had competition.

"Pete normally kicks off the cleaning run about nine. The usual deal is an hour per day, five days a week and you may as well start tomorrow."

"I'll be here at nine then."

Bob was already standing at the door watching perfect little waves run down the left hand point. He took some money from his pocket. "Righto Sally, here's two week's rent. We need to snap into action as the day is gettin' on. We've got the shack to set up and we might even get a late arvo surf if we're lucky... Yooooohhhhh!" he hooted like a teenager, throwing a tube riding stance under the doorway.

The lads took off to investigate their new home. There were various camps dotted along the hillside and in behind the dunes closer to the ocean. The shacks were simple, rough-built dwellings, made from rocks, timber and by the looks of it, whatever else was lying around.

Bob brought Freedom to a stop outside a cute little shack behind the dunes, partly shaded by two trees. Eagerly they both jumped out like kids heading for an ice cream truck. The previous times Bob had been here, he'd never stayed in the love shack and was frothing to say the least. As they approached the front door, the fun and games continued. It was a laughing wrestle to see who could get inside first.

It was one big room with different sections for cooking, eating, sleeping etc. The side closest to the ocean was open with a verandah, which then led out onto a narrow track between the dunes and straight onto the beach. From the track, there was a perfect view of the point. Dave became silent again as he stood there with Bob watching three perfect waves rolling through, and there were only two other surfers in the water.

"Let's leave the set-up for tomorrow," Bob said, quickly receiving a big nod and a smile from Dave.

They surfed until sunset and in the end it was only the two of them out there. There was the odd head high set and Dave was in his element. He was feeling vital and clear. Bob schooled him on the reef and which waves to look for. The trickiest part was getting in and out of the water, due to the sharp rocks. Patience was the real key there.

The following morning dawned another joyous day. A strong, icy offshore was blowing, straight off the desert. Dave rugged up and made sure he was on time for his first day of work.

"Good morning. You must be Dave," Pete said in a cheery voice, shaking his hand.

"Pleased to meet you," Dave replied, getting all official to impress the new boss. They were standing next to an old Holden ute that was looking very much like the work truck.

"Jump in mate, let's do it. Might not even be an hour today as the camp's so quiet. The swell's jacked a bit too, and once that wind eases up, it'll be pumpin'!" he said, with a twinkle in his eye.

Pete was short like Sally but he was a real nugget.

Broad shoulders and very strong looking, with a happy face, weathered by the desert sun and winds. He was very interested in Dave's life and where he'd come from. It turned out Pete was originally from Sydney as well and twenty years ago had stumbled upon this place and never left. He spoke slowly and had loads of funny stories.

Pete parked the ute on some rocky ground, not too far from the love shack.

"How about you collect the rubbish from this section," Pete said, handing Dave a bunch of replacement bags. "And I'll go sort this dunny out. Don't want to throw ya straight in the deep end on day one!"

"Not gunna argue with ya there," Dave replied with a laugh, taking off on his mission. It was an easy job and quite social as well. As he entered one of the camps, a beautiful, blonde-haired woman came out to greet him: "Hello. I have some more here, before you take it," she said, in a foreign accent. Dave's heart skipped a beat.

"No worries," he replied, letting out a nervous laugh. She moved in close and filled the bag a little more. This woman smelt good. "Is your name Grace?" he inquired, putting the pieces of the puzzle together and tying the bag off.

"Yes, that's right."

"Oh great. Sally told me to come and see you."

"Really," she said, looking into his eye's.

"Yeah... About using your spare massage table."

From behind her caravan popped another woman, who looked like she was on a mission. "Good morning," she said, acknowledging them both. "Okay Grace, you ready for this walk or what?"

"Yes, ready to go," Grace replied, a little rattled by her friend and not wanting to keep her waiting. "Listen, um, what was your name?"

"It's Dave."

"Listen Dave, I can't talk now, but how about you come over for a cup of tea after lunch."

"Okay, I'll see you then."

The hour passed by quickly and as Pete had predicted, the wind was dropping out. The waves at the point were looking epic. Dave arrived back to camp and there was a note from Bob on the table:

Gone surfin... see ya out there!

Dave grabbed his board, bag of gear and began the walk out to the point. There were already ten guys in the line-up and they were catching some beauties. Dave felt no need to rush today. He enjoyed the walk, the sounds, and stopped to talk with a few people on the track. The slower pace of life had begun back at Bob's brother's place and it was continuing to grow every day.

I wonder how relaxed I could possibly get? he thought, stopping for a moment. He took a deep breath in, looked around and was hypnotised by the beauty surrounding him, the raw nature, the glistening ocean. *What if life really could be this easy and fun?*

The surf was all-time. At one stage, a pod of dolphins came through the break and Dave jumped off his board to get as close as he could. He loved the sounds they made underwater and the smiles they brought to everyone's faces. Pete joined them in the surf and he was by far the stand-out performer. Just about every wave he caught was from further up the point than anyone else and he got tubed on each one of them. He had the place totally wired. That's what twenty years of practice does!

Throughout the morning, Dave had been thinking of Grace and was quite nervous about going to see her after lunch. There was something about her he couldn't put his finger on. She was twice his age but the way he felt when he met her was amazing. The afternoon came around quickly. When the time was right he gathered all his new-found confidence and courage together and went to see her. Bob teased him as he headed out the door: "Good luck on your first date mate!" Dave had no reply except a cheeky, nervous smile.

A few moments later, he was standing in front of her door.

"Hello, anyone home?"

"Yes, come in," came a sweet but strong voice, making the hairs on Dave's arms stand up. Grace had an elaborate set-up consisting of a caravan and a huge annexe. Half the annexe had been separated with sheets and sarongs and he could see part of a massage table in there.

"Come up Dave, I'm in the van."

"Wow! It's great in here." He looked around in wonder, opening the flywire door. It was how he'd imagined a gypsy's caravan to be. There were lots of red and maroon cushions and colourful sarongs hanging from the walls. Her bed looked fit for a queen. It felt homely and very alive. Grace even had a proper antique style tea pot and mugs to match, all set out on the table.

"Welcome to my desert home," she said proudly, before getting up and giving Dave a deep, warm hug. *This is a next-level hug*, he thought to himself, feeling the warmth of her belly pressing firmly against his. He could feel electricity shooting through his body and began getting an erection. He pulled away awkwardly and sat down as quickly as possible so she wouldn't notice the growing lump in his board shorts.

"Would you like some tea?" Grace offered warmly, sitting down across from him.

"Sure, I'd love some thanks," came the reply from a now more at ease young man, knowing his secret was safe.

In front of Dave on the wall, were two artistic pictures of naked men and women making love, painted in such a surreal way that it gave him another dose of discomfort. He pulled himself together, quickly.

"I was wondering Grace, if you're not using your spare massage table up in the office, if I could use it? I need to make a few extra bucks and was thinkin' a couple of massages here and there could do the trick."

"I would love to be your first customer," she announced in her thick, Dutch accent. "My lower back has been giving me trouble and I need some healing there... what do you know about massage?"

Dave laughed. "Not much at all to be honest, but I figured I'd just learn as I go."

"Really?" came her cute, mocking reply. "Okay, I've got an idea. How about we meet in here for an hour each day around this time. One day you will give me a massage and the following day I will do some healing work on you and I can train you as we go... how does that sound?"

"That sounds too good to be true. It would've been a bit dodgy me startin' out not havin' a clue anyway, so I'd be stoked to accept your offer." He lifted up his full cup of tea towards Grace. "Cheers!" he said with a smile, the fine china clinking together.

11. DESERT GRACE

"What sort of healing work do you do exactly?" he asked Grace, taking a sip of tea.

"Well, these days I call myself a 'Sacred Sexual Healer' or 'Dakini'. I travel the world helping people to heal their guilt, shame and fear around sexuality and help encourage them to really step into their power. It's controversial work but very worthwile."

It seemed to Dave that Grace had just grown bigger and become very radiant. He wasn't sure at all how to take what she'd just said and sat there, not saying a word. Discomfort filled the van. Grace felt it worthwhile to explain a little more.

"When I was about your age, I started out doing bodywork and massage on sports teams in Holland with a big company who also trained me. I then studied counselling and various holistic therapies and eventually reached the conclusion that I needed to work in the field of sexuality. It is an area of healing that is often overlooked. Our sexual energy is our life force and if that's repressed or blocked in any way, we are not even living half the life we are capable of living."

Dave was absorbing her words like a giant sponge. His mind slowly dropped the idea that he was about to be locked into a gypsy's caravan and turned into a desert sex slave and he loosened up a bit. It was weird though, 'cause part of him liked the idea! She was in fact, quite an exotic woman and he felt attracted to her. No one had ever spoken to him so openly about sex before, not even Anne. Intrigue was growing and so was that lump in his pants again!

"It's especially important for young people like yourself to learn to be comfortable with your sexuality and energy. Unfortunately these days, we are educated by disrespectful pornography and awkward parents. One of the most important aspects of life is barely even talked about! It is changing in Europe though, but ever so slowly."

She was right on the money. Dave had watched a lot of porn movies and it was endless as to what was available on the Internet – from violent fucking through to sex with innocent young kids and everything in between. Dave and his mates were always showing each other new stuff and making jokes about it. Sometimes though, it made him feel sick. As far as sex went: for him it was always an uncertain, intense event that was usually over before it had barely begun. He'd only ever had sex with two women before and for the last two years it had only been with Anne.

Grace gently put her cup back down on the table and leaned forward a little, exposing her cleavage.

"You know, in some ancient tribes your very first sexual experience was a sacred 'Rite Of Passage'. A ceremony that marked a turning point in your life. It was undertaken with awareness, respect and love. How about for you? How was your first sexual experience?"

Dave was surprised with her question and felt hesitant to go there. *What am I even doin' here talkin' about sex with this woman?* he thought, looking down into his cup of tea, shaking his head. "You really wanna know?"

"Yes, but only if you're okay with it."

"Well... there definitely wasn't awareness, respect or love, that's for sure!" he laughed, looking up a Grace. "It was in the back of a car outside a party. I was sixteen and that drunk I don't even really remember what happened. It was with one of my mates older sisters, who was pretty experienced... at least that's what she thought at the time! I do remember it was super uncomfortable though and I got a wild cramp in my leg. Oohh, that's right... Not long after, she went back into the same car with some other guy, which didn't leave me feelin' too good. I was stoked to have had sex but it was a bit of a let down to be honest."

"I'd say you're not the only one with that sort of story." Grace said, finishing her cup of tea.

"Yeah, I guess that's true," he said, relieved.

"So… let's get started. I am ready for my massage!" she said in a cheeky tone, standing up from the table.

Dave was caught by surprise. *This woman knows what she wants*, he thought, while studying her cute, little pot belly poking out from under her mid-riff top. Dave was in no space to question this woman and was now safe to stand, as his erection had totally vanished. "Okay, let's do it!" he replied, with fresh enthusiasm.

The massage room was also set up beautifully and Grace wasted no time in stripping all her gear off and lying down face first on the table, as though she'd done it plenty of times before. Dave totally froze and didn't quite know what to do. He could feel his cock growing rapidly in his shorts again… *What does this woman really want from me? We've only just met! Does she want more than just a massage?* His mind was racing out of control and he could feel his heart beating a million miles per hour. By now his erection was so hard it could've cut a diamond in half. He quickly tucked it up into the top of his shorts to not be caught out and just stood there like one of those plastic manikins in a clothes store.

Sensing his shock, Grace spoke up: "Relax Dave, this is your first lesson. To be comfortable around a naked body. Take a deep breath in and feel your feet on the ground. We are all born like this you know!" she joked. "The oil is there on the table and my lower back is ready for your healing hands."

Relax! Are you serious? He'd only just met this

woman fifteen minutes ago and there she was, lying totally naked in front of him. He was extremely uncomfortable, but a small part of him was also up for the challenge. He decided to take Grace's advice and took a couple of deep breaths. This helped iron out the wobbles and he lightened up a bit.

"Okay, the breath thing seems to have worked. I just wasn't expecting this to be the first lesson though," he said, letting out another nervous chuckle.

"I understand, and it's okay. Whatever is happening for you, just allow it. I am more than ready for your healing hands now," came Grace's reassuring words from under the table.

She certainly had a beautiful body... A real, curvy, middle aged woman's body. And there she was laying right in front of him in all her magnificence. It was awe inspiring! Dave studied her lines and the texture of her skin. Apart from Anne, he hadn't been around a naked woman before. It was beginning to feel good. Dave took another deep breath and reached for the oil.

He rubbed some on his hands and began. *I wonder if that's where she wants it? Is that enough oil?* he thought, tentatively rubbing her back and starting to feel the muscles along each side of the spine. Her skin felt soft and silky and there were all these tiny little blond hairs. There was no way in the world his erection was going to disappear now. Blood was pumping through his whole body and his palms were red hot. Grace was delighted with his touch and gave him some tips as he went.

"That's it... that flowing motion you've got, that's great... oooohh yes... that part there... ooohhh... can you just hold that?" It was almost too much for Dave. Grace's moans took him over the edge. He zoned out and thought of his friends back in the city. *Imagine if they could see me now. In paradise, massaging a naked, Dutch cougar!*

"Stay present Dave. Breathe... feel your feet and be in your hands." *How did she know I drifted off? This woman is tuned,* he thought and took another deep breath. He was beginning to enjoy himself and it seemed the more he was enjoying it, the more Grace was enjoying it.

"You're picking it up well... Next I would love it if you massage my legs and ass."

"That'd be my pleasure," Dave responded, in an overly confident way, trying to hide the fact he was being stretched again.

Dave poured some more oil onto his hands and began on Grace's legs. Her calves were strong and tight and were definitely needing some work. He realised if he went too deep, too soon, her body would just tense up, so he had to work in gently to get a good release. She had beautiful long legs and Dave slowly, but surely, moved up towards her ass. By now he was more relaxed again and starting to realise just how good this whole situation was.

He eventually reached her bum, which was extra soft and a bit wobbly but he didn't hold back at all. It was fun and weird at the same time. Grace continued moaning and making a lot of noise as her muscles relaxed. She opened her legs just slightly, appearing to get comfortable and Dave got a full view of her vagina. This took his breath away... it was a sight to behold! He saw her lips, all the different colours... he could even smell her. He was being hypnotised and his cock was now hard again.

Out of the blue Grace rolled over, exposing the front of her body to him. This time she caught his eye:

"Lesson two... eye contact with a beautiful naked woman, with no alcohol," she said, in her very sexy style. Dave laughed awkwardly and took another breath:

"I'm enjoyin' your lessons. I've never been to a school like this before."

"Well, it sounds like you're ready for lesson three then. I want you to massage my breasts!" she suggested assertively.

By now his secret was totally out of the bag, he could no longer hide it. His face had gone bright red and he was starting to sweat, as Grace had full vision of the hard mountain in his shorts. Dave didn't know whether to run or hide.

"Could be time to breathe again," she said, in a relaxed manner. "If at any time this is too much for you, you can stop, you know. I am not forcing you into anything here. This is exactly what I was talking about before. Since when did a handsome young man such as yourself, learn to be afraid of his erection? This is your manhood, your power! How would it be for you to be comfortable with that? Men spend their youth fearing their erections and their old age fearing not getting one. It's very strange."

Ninety five percent of Dave wanted to get the hell out of there but the remaining five percent was totally intrigued and he longed to be at ease with all parts of himself in any situation... so he stayed. There was that much happening for him his mind completely shut off and tears began welling up in his eyes. He'd realised, most of his life he'd thought that his penis was wrong, too small or it needed to be hidden away, especially if it was hard. There he stood in front of Grace, exposed and melting. Tears came from deep within him and streamed down his face.

"It's all okay Dave. Just let it come," she reassured him, sitting up on the edge of the table. "All is welcome here."

She softly approached him and put her arms out for a hug. All Dave wanted to do was get away. He resisted the embrace a few moments and then crumbled, receiving her warmth. The crying deepened and tears rolled down her naked back. He was torn open and Grace just held him, in a strong, yet loving way. Eventually the tears faded and were replaced by an overwhelming sense of peace. It was by far the longest hug Dave had ever shared. When he was ready, he pulled away and looked directly at Grace, slightly uneasy, realising she was still unclothed.

"Thanks for your support," he said quietly, looking deeply into her soft, blue eyes.

"Well... we didn't quite get to lesson three," she replied in her cheeky style, laughing again. "But my feeling is, this will do for the day. How are you going?"

"Yeah, okay. I'm pretty wobbly but the fact I'm standin' here, kind of not worried and you're still naked in front of me, feels different. It's hard to say, but I feel more relaxed in my body or somethin'." Grace slipped her clothes back on without much fuss and sat back up on the table.

"What happened just then Dave, was really special and it's exactly the work that I do. I help people to realise they are absolutely perfect as they are, and once that process begins, the guilt, shame and fear they have been holding is revealed and starts to fall away. It normally takes a few sessions before the releasing begins… I guess, today you were ready. You are an amazing young man! Thank you for your courage."

"This is all so new to me. The last month of my life has been bizarre. Almost like I'm on another planet and it just keeps gettin' wilder and wilder. Like just what happened now, is so far from what I've known, that my mind just freaks out and goes blank. All I want to do is escape but there is a small part of me that keeps me here because it knows it's exactly what I need… it's really weird."

He sat up on the table alongside Grace, becoming more and more comfortable each moment. She responded warmly, putting her hand lightly on his thigh. "It's a very powerful time to be alive Dave. Those of us on the planet now have chosen to be here for a very special reason. We are moving from the old world of fear into a new way of living that is grounded in love, gratitude, ease and joy… and that is exciting."

She paused. "All the ancient cultures have predicted it and it's actually happening right now!" They were looking each other straight in the eyes and Dave felt goose bumps all over his body. He wondered: *am I actually part of this change?* As if Grace had heard his thoughts, she went on:

"And guess what: you and I and everyone on the planet are part of it. We all have our role to play and the sooner we begin living from our hearts, the sooner we will all see that heaven on earth is already right here, right now." Dave's mind had shut off again. *Living from the heart? Heaven on earth? Was Grace an undercover religious nut out to brain wash him?* So many questions flooded his mind and the alarm bells to get out of there were suddenly ringing more loudly than ever.

"Listen Grace, I gotta go," he said frankly, heading for the door without turning back.

"I'll see you tomorrow Dave, thanks for the massage. It was fantastic!"

12. ENERGY PUMP

Dave barely heard her and was so relieved to be out of that tent. The sun, the fresh air, the trees around him... *There's no way I'm going back to see her. That woman is off her head!* he reasoned, wondering how he'd even allowed himself to get into that situation in the first place.

All he could think of now was jumping into the ocean. He found a new track over the sand dunes he hadn't seen before, took off his shirt and headed straight for the sparkling water. The wind had changed slightly and the waves on the point were looking average, but it was still a magical day and the sun warmed his face and chest.

He immersed himself into the ocean and instantly, his whole body was at ease. Dave was at home in the water. It was very healing for him. As he walked back up the beach, he stopped and lay down flat on his back, surrendering to the day and began reflecting on his time with Grace. He flashed on a memory of when he was much younger and his parents had caught him masturbating in his bedroom. Dave had felt guilty and wrong and had barely even done it again since then. He also saw clearly how frustrated he was when he had sex and couldn't do it as well as the porn stars. He glimpsed on just how awkward he really was with his sexuality and got more of an understanding of the work Grace was doing. The afternoon sun had by now warmed his whole body and he drifted off to sleep.

It was almost sunset before Dave awoke and the desert chill was moving in for the evening. He hurried back to the shack to get warm. Bob had prepared a delicious dinner of fresh fish and was curious about what Dave had been up to.

"Pretty long first date my friend. How'd it all go?" he asked inquisitively.

"Far out... I don't even know where to start!" Dave replied, taking a seat at the table and sharing breath for breath what had happened. Bob listened closely and loved every minute of the story.

"Is she very busy?" he jumped in, as soon as Dave had finished. "I'd love to make a booking," he said and then let go into one of his raucous full belly laughs. Dave had no choice but to join in. It was refreshing to see the funny side. There was still no way he was going back though.

The next day dawned and the morning was an exact replica of the day before. Dave enjoyed his work with Pete, especially hearing a load of tall stories from back in the days. Pete also shared some advice about the best waves to pick out at the point, and where the most makeable tube sections were. Dave listened intently 'cause he'd seen Pete in action and was well impressed.

Walking back from his mid-morning surf, Dave started feeling pulled to go and see Grace again. All morning he'd been clear and quite relieved about not going, but now this five percent of him was getting in the way again.

It's my turn to receive today and my shoulders could really use a massage. That could be the way to do it, he thought, stopping on the track and looking back to see a set roll through the point. *So that's it. I'll just be clear with her and ask for a shoulder massage only.*

"Come on in Dave," came Grace's sexy voice as he slipped in through the annexe door. "I was not so sure if I'd see you today and I am very happy you have come." She came out of the van and met him in the annexe to share a hug. Dave's fears of why or why not he should have come, fell away in her soft embrace. She smelt soooo good and the hug seemed to go on even longer than the day before.

"My shoulders are cooked from all the surfin' and I'm wonderin' if you could massage them today?" He began, trying his hardest to be clear and assertive.

"That's a great idea, and a perfect place to start," Grace replied.

They both stepped into the massage room. Dave slipped his shirt off and double-checked that his shorts were firmly tied up. He'd worn his draw-string-numbers to ensure they stayed on! He lay face down on the table and Grace began to weave her magic. Her touch was gentle yet deep and his shoulders were celebrating. She taught him to breathe through the painful spots to help them release. He eventually fully relaxed and the hour was over before he knew it.

A week passed and Dave was thoroughly enjoying his daily sessions with Grace. She would be leaving in six days and he'd decided to soak up as much knowledge from her while he had the opportunity. It was now, without a doubt, the highlight of his day, especially when the surf had gone flat. Grace's back was much better thanks to Dave's improving massage skills and he'd even successfully passed lesson three. It hadn't stopped there though and he was now up to lesson seven! Bob loved hearing about his daily adventures and had his own insights to give in certain areas.

One night at a full moon party on the beach, the three of them went skinny dipping together along with a few other friends. It was a huge step for Dave and he felt so liberated afterwards. The work he'd been doing with Grace was paying off and he was beginning to feel more and more at home with all parts of his body. That night he'd stepped over the line and the following day when he lay down to receive from Grace, he was naked.

"I am not sure what lesson we are up to, but we could be ticking another one off today!" she laughed. "I will be working on your lower back, hips and ass, as it seems that's what you are wanting."

"Perfect," came the tranquil voice from under the massage table.

"And remember," she continued, "if at any stage it's too much or you want me to stop, please let me know."

He was feeling very open and trusting around Grace now. All his fears had gone out the window. She began on his bum and he tensed up, not expecting it so soon.

"This ass has not seen a lot of sun," she played, running her palms firmly across his pale backside.

"It's true, but it's now seen some moonlight!" came the voice from under the table again. Dave wanted to continue talking but she'd hit a spot that sent pain flying through his entire body.

"Just breathe, like I taught you. Right down into my hands... that's good... We hold so much in our hips and ass. Just allow it to melt..." It was a cross between pleasure and pain and all Dave could do was keep breathing. She began massaging down into the back of his balls and groin which made him jump.

"It is okay, breathe Dave. Allow it all... and remember, let me know if it's too much." Dave shuffled around a little, lifting his hips to make room for his erection and rested back down to enjoy the ride.

Grace continued even to the point of reaching in past his balls and rubbing the back of his hard penis with her soft, oily hand.

"Feel this energy growing in you... this is your primal power. You can use this energy to create the life of your dreams. It is essential for you to honour and master this part of yourself if you want to live to your full potential."

Dave was exploding with life. He felt as though he was hooked up to a power plant or lightning had hit him. He was fully 'turned on' and breathing and relaxing at the same time. He'd glimpsed on this when he was drunk but it was never so clear and strong.

"Now for today's lesson!" Grace declared with excitement, totally present and energised herself. "I want you to turn over and I will teach you the art of drawing up your energy." Dave was in heaven and did exactly as instructed.

Wow... I've come a long way in a week, he thought to himself, now on his back, fully erect and totally exposed to Grace.

"Feel this muscle in here," she said, pressing firmly between the back of his balls and his anus. "This is your energy pump. And when the energy gets too strong down here," she continued, gently massaging his balls, "or when you feel close to ejaculation, you need to squeeze this muscle and breathe in, drawing the energy up the back of your spine and into your head... try that first." Dave squeezed his ass muscle and took a deep breath in through his nose, visualising the energy going up his back. His head began to tingle. It was working!

"Next, you press the top of your tongue against the roof of your mouth. Not just behind the teeth but right up on the roof."

"Cool, I got it" he said, with a funny sort of tongue-in-the-way accent.

"As you breathe out, totally relax and let the energy go down the front of your body into your belly, your power centre. Do this a few times."

Dave had never felt so much freedom around his sexuality and was quickly falling in love with this Dutch Goddess. How could he not? Especially while she was standing there, caressing his balls! She barely even looked forty, was energised, healthy and super-interesting. He remembered what he was doing and breathed the energy up a few more times, squeezing his ass muscle as tightly as he could. His erection began to shrink a little.

"Okay, great, looks like you're getting it. The whole reason I'm teaching you this," she paused, putting one hand on his heart, "is to give you a tool you can use for your whole life whether you are making love or self-pleasuring. The ancient Chinese believed that when men ejaculate, they lose much of their essence or life force and if you want to age with vitality, it's healthy to practise these techniques and not waste your semen recklessly. At your age though, you are at your sexual peak and have so much energy, that if you ejaculated every day it probably wouldn't even affect you. We are all unique beings though, so it's fantastic to experiment and see what works best." Grace moved away from him to put some more oil on her hands.

"The idea is to bring yourself close to ejaculation but to stop before you crest over. If you practise by pleasuring yourself with oil in the morning and get close to the point of no return two or three times, the energy you create and can use in your day, is phenomenal. To have control of your ejaculation is a long-lost secret and once you master it, your whole world will be transformed... but like anything, it takes practice.

"It's important you don't get too much energy stuck in your head though. So remember to put your tongue on the roof and breathe it down. Worst case scenario: if there's too much energy and you're uncomfortable, just ejaculate to release the pressure. It's a lot of trial and error at first and as you increase your energy and pleasure threshold your body actually starts rewiring itself. Previously blocked channels open throughout your energetic system and you begin to become more and more orgasmic every day."

Dave was drinking all this in, totally drunk with lust. Grace continued: "Some people find they can breathe the energy up and out the top of their heads and then as they breathe out they visualise the energy passing out through their feet and into the earth. The basic key for moving energy is breath, sound and movement. Especially for men, to grunt and groan and thrash around wildly can be really helpful to get things moving." Grace was now rubbing his thighs strongly and was checking in with herself to see if she'd left anything out and her sweet voice began again, combined with that cheeky smile: "How would it be for you Dave, to be sexually self-sufficient and to master your ejaculation?"

"It would change my life for sure. With my last girlfriend I would always come very quickly and I'd even thought about tryin' some of that stuff they advertise to make you last longer. My mate tried it though and didn't rate it at all. He said it was like a bad acid trip!"

"Plus, that is only a quick fix. You know what the greatest thing about learning these techniques is? Eventually you can orgasm without ejaculating. And the orgasm is not just like a little sneeze when you ejaculate now but it becomes a full body experience that is extremely blissful and very life-giving."

Dave was ecstatic and loved the idea. He reached down to hold his balls and penis and then rubbed his hands over his body. His erection had returned and a strong desire was growing in him to have sex with Grace. He fantasised, *would that be the next lesson?* but at this stage did not have the courage to ask. She was looking sexier every moment and it was almost getting too much for him. He sat up and grabbed Grace's arm, pulling her close to him. Nature had taken over and his mind had disappeared once again.

They were eye to eye now, and Dave pulled her in even closer. He motioned to kiss her but she gently eased away from him. He pulled her in close once again and this time Grace reacted more strongly, freeing herself from his grip.

"I will not do this Dave. I am not available for a romantic relationship with you. I know today's session has gone to the next level but this is all about you, not me. This energy you are feeling right now is very powerful and you must learn to get comfortable with it yourself first, before sharing it with others." Dave was now bright red in the face and feeling really stupid. His energy had totally shifted, he felt two foot tall. "I'm sorry... I understand. I was at boiling point and all I wanted was to have sex with you, like I was on auto-pilot or something."

"Please, do not see this as wrong. Your energy is so alive and beautiful but I have boundaries in my work so I need to be clear with you and look after my needs. Don't worry though, you are young and handsome and still have many women to pleasure."

The two of them hugged and Dave suddenly found the whole thing amusing and began laughing wildly at himself, at the whole situation. Grace caught the flame and their bellies danced together. Dave's sexual energy had found an outlet and the two of them hugged and laughed for what seemed like an eternity.

13. DOLPHIN JOY

"Okay... NOW!" Dave said, and they all tossed the colourful array of flowers across Grace's windscreen as she pulled out of camp with her big gypsy caravan in tow. Grace leaned out the window, surprised and unable to see clearly where she was going.

"Thank you! Have a blissful life Dave and always remember your amazingness!" she said excitedly. The words anchored directly into Dave's heart and triggered a wave of tears. He'd helped her pack up slowly the previous couple of days and really thought he'd be ready for this moment. He wasn't sure if they were tears of sadness, gratitude or joy.

He'd rounded up Bob and a few friends to surprise Grace with a 'flower shower', as she was leaving. It was the least he could do for all that she had shared with him. His world was quickly expanding and Grace had helped rocket him to a new level.

Bob came over and gave him a reassuring hug: "You alright little bro?"

Dave stood there crying and uncertain as the caravan disappeared over the hill. "That woman changed my life," he declared, pulling himself together a little.

"Yep, women tend to do that."

They walked slowly back to the love shack in silence. Dave felt as though a piece of him had left with Grace. There was now so much sadness moving through him it was overwhelming and he didn't know which way to turn.

"I need to be alone. I'm goin' for a walk," he said, holding another flood of tears back.

Bob could feel the tension building up in his young friend. "Okay bro. Now could be a good time to use those tools I taught you. Remember, if anger's there, you can beat the sand or do those hand screams. And for sadness, pull your arms back and expose your heart. They are just emotions man — energy in motion — they will move. If you need any support or a listening ear, you know I'm here too," Bob finished compassionately. Dave looked him in the eye, still managing to hold back the impending flood.

"Thanks, I know," he said and continued out the door, heading towards the ocean.

The feelings were intensifying rapidly and he walked quickly up the beach to get to a place where he could open the floodgates safely without freaking out any of the other campers. The walk became a run and tears started falling. There was a rock up ahead that offered some sanctuary. He fell to his knees behind it and crumbled onto the sand, crying, gasping for breath, chest burning.

"WHY DID SHE LEAVE ME??" he screamed loudly and began bashing the sand violently with his fists. "HOW COULD SHE DO IT!!" A thunderstorm of anger exploded through his body. Dave thrashed about like an attacking crocodile, totally out of control. "RRRRRHHHHHHHH... FUCK YOU!!! I HATE YOU!!! WHY DID YOU DO THIS TO ME!!!"

He went on screaming and beating the sand until his voice had vanished. Eventually the storm passed and he collapsed onto his back, exhausted, dripping with sweat, his body electrified and shaky.

He'd now moved into the centre of the cyclone and there was this absolute stillness and calm that he wasn't expecting. His emotions had gone from one extreme to the other and he just lay there, totally silent in the morning sun. After a while, the ocean was calling and he pulled off his sandy, sweat soaked shirt and walked down to the water. Diving in was orgasmic, his body felt so alive. The sensation of the water on his skin was pure, outrageous joy.

Walking back home, he felt like a new man. He wondered how long all that anger and sadness had been inside him and if there was any more left. The emotions that had just come up though, didn't even feel relevant to Grace leaving. It was as if her departure had triggered a switch inside him and everything had just burst forth from there. It was kinda scary!

If I keep that up they'll throw me in the nut house for sure, he thought, followed by a little chuckle. He reflected on how kids throw tantrums when they're upset and then a few minutes later they're all happy and light again. *It would be a different world if everyone carried on like that.*

It was the weekend, so Dave had the full day to himself. No work, no session with Grace. What the hell was he going to do? The waves were still tiny, so a surf was out of the question as well. He'd been longing to go on a walk south of the point that Bob had been raving about. Maybe today was the day. Bob reckoned there were all these natural crystal formations set up in a circle and that it was apparently some ancient ceremonial site. Arriving back at the shack, he surprised his friend, who was just rolling out his yoga mat.

"You amped for a walk today?" he asked.

"Woah! You're lookin' better man. Sounds like you sure let out some demons down there... well done! How'd ya go with the tools?"

"Yeah good, they definitely helped me move it all through, that's for sure. I felt so clear and quiet afterwards, it was kinda strange."

"Man... that silence you felt, that spaciousness. That's who you truly are. So often our busy minds and sticky emotions get in the way of drinkin' that nectar. I'm really stoked you got a taste." Bob was staring right at Dave with his big eyes and smile going on. He backed off and lay down on his mat. "I'm gunna stretch it up a little now but I'm feelin' today's a perfect day for a stroll. I'd love to join you. How 'bout we cruise in an hour or so?"

"Sounds great. I need some muesli anyway, I'm starvin'."

Dave went and sat up on the track overlooking the ocean to have breakfast. He reflected on the morning's events and became aware that underneath the lingering droplets of shakiness, he felt clear, confident and powerful. He wondered if this was the 'amazingness' that Grace was speaking of? It was as though he didn't need any confirmation from anyone for anything and that was empowering. The energy and aliveness he was carrying brought a big smile to his face. Sitting there, having his muesli, he felt like he had all the time in the world.

The hour flew by. They packed a few essentials for the walk and were off. The camp was very quiet today and they didn't see a soul walking out to the point. Once around the corner and heading south, it was like they'd entered another world. The landscape was made up of rugged, broken cliffs and rock formations that had been battered by relentless ocean swells for thousands of years. It looked prehistoric and very different from the bay where the camp was. The ocean was almost dead flat and the wind was light. For a change there was barely a sound.

They walked for over an hour in silence, occasionally

acknowledging each other but generally just keeping to themselves. A couple of times a large eagle had flown past. Dave felt his whole body starting to relax more and more. It had been a huge morning emotionally and it was such a blessing to have some time to integrate everything. Dave also felt having Bob there on the walk with him gave him security and support. A deeper sense of ease continued to grow inside him.

After climbing some huge sand dunes that almost came right out of the ocean, they walked further south to the area which contained the crystals. It was extraordinary. A half open cave, about the size of two cars, containing well over a hundred, vertical, clear quartz crystals rising up out of the rock in a ring formation. In the middle was a flat area, made up of black shiny rock. Bob headed straight for the centre, took off his pack and lay down.

"This place is soooo healing man," he shared with Dave. "I got busted up a few years ago on a big swell at the point and really hurt my back, almost couldn't walk for a few days. Once I became a little more mobile a good friend brought me here, and he had me lay down like this for hours. When I eventually got up the pain had completely vanished. I was blown away! Apparently the sun warmed rock and the energy of these crystals has extraordinary powers. It's a very sacred place and he reckons the Aboriginal people used it for that very reason for thousands of years."

Dave's whole body had turned to goose bumps. He could definitely feel this was a very special place.

He also put his bag down and stepped into the circle to lay next to Bob. The warmth of the rock on his back and legs began easing his muscles.

"Thanks for bringing me here," he said, dissolving more and more into the rock. They both lay there and automatically went back into silence mode. Dave's body felt really heavy, like he was being pulled into the earth, so relaxing... Time slipped away and he actually fell asleep. Bob heard him snoring a couple of times and found it quite amusing.

Eventually Bob made a move to get up. This woke Dave, who didn't have a clue where he was at first but slowly pieced it all together. His face felt dry and a his body was very hot, like he'd been slowly cooked in an oven. Dave downed half a bottle of well needed water and instantly felt more alive. It was well after lunch time and the food they'd brought along didn't last five minutes.

Again, not a lot was said and they peacefully made their way back to camp, arriving just as the sun was setting. It had been a different kind of day. Very quiet and reflective, and also extremely healing. Dave was knackered and after a light dinner went straight to bed.

The following morning he rose early, and walked outside in the pre-dawn light to check the surf. There wasn't much wind and the swell had come up overnight. The waves looked great and he was really keen to go out. Dave was full of beans after a long night's sleep and wasted no time in having a quick feed, gathering his gear and heading out to the point. He was pumped!

There was already one guy in the water and the ocean was like glass. Hardly a breath of wind. It was also bigger than he'd originally thought, with the odd four-footer peeling off. Dave threw his wettie on, waxed up and got out there. His surf fitness was back; it was like he'd never stopped. He caught wave after wave and even negotiated his way through a few nice tubes, following Pete's advice on which waves to pick.

At one point a huge pod of dolphins came through the line up. As usual, Dave jumped off his board and swam down to greet them. He was addicted to their whistle and the clicking sounds of their sonar. As he popped up to get some air, a beautiful wave approached. Climbing back onto his board, he swung around and with a few strong paddles, he was on. From the word go he knew this would be another tube ride... the wave was looking so clean and perfect.

He drew a cruisey bottom turn and pulled up into the hollow part of the wave. To his surprise, riding alongside him inside the wave was a dolphin. The wave threw out over him, and there he was, flying along, inside a watery, crystal cavern with a huge dolphin barely thirty centimetres away, travelling at exactly the same speed. If he'd reached out he could have touched it. Suddenly the wave changed and water sprayed across his face. He temporarily lost sight of his new friend but managed to stay on his board and feel his way out of the tube.

He rode the wave till the end, totally stoked. He

pulled off and sat on his board in wonder. *That's gotta be the highlight of my surfing career so far!* he thought, in full bliss mode. Then, to his surprise, the dolphin popped up right beside him, wanting to play some more. It looked straight at him with so much love, joy and acceptance in its eyes that Dave's heart blew open. In its own way, the dolphin was talking with him.

"WOW!!! That was fun. Do you want to do it again?" he asked, looking straight back into the dolphin's eyes. The dolphin bobbed up and down gazing at him, not even a metre from his knee. Dave was sure it was smiling at him. Then, it sank down under his board and popped up on the other side. This was crazy! He wasn't sure if it had been ten seconds or two minutes... his mind now totally out to lunch. This sort of thing is not in the text book of life and eventually Dave started to freak out – it was getting far too strange! As soon as the dolphin sensed the fear, it was gone, disappearing back into the deep blue ocean.

Dave continued to sit there on his board, in a daze. Once the fear vanished, he felt drunk with love and completely overwhelmed. The way that dolphin had looked straight through him... he couldn't even begin to describe the feeling.

That afternoon, he knew he had to write all this down, so he dug out the book Denise had given him that was still a virgin. He found his pen and decided to christen the book with a poem. He hadn't written one since high school, but if his writing career was ever going to start again then today was the day.

14. MAKARA

Divine Dolphin Love
Gratefulness pours from my being.
The ocean, the sun, the space.
I am immersed in her healing womb.
Playfulness explodes.
I am eight years old again.
Then they appear,
A family of messiahs from their watery realm.
They have come to ride the swells with the surfers.
My heart explodes, excitement rises.
A deep peace resonates.
I stroke into a peeling left hander.
Slowly off the bottom and into the hook.
There, right beside me is my new friend.
Together we slide through space and time.
We enter another realm.

The love, the joy, the ecstasy, the connection,
Pouring from us both.
This is a meeting of hearts.
The wave passes and there we are.
New friends, celebrating and sharing the bliss of being alive right now.

Dave shared his experience with Bob, who was also blown away and spoke up excitedly:

"This has so much significance man. I'm gunna do some research this arvo and see what I can come up with." He walked out to the van and returned with a box of old books. Dave was also proud of his poem and read it out loud to Bob, who loved it and encouraged him to write more.

"That's awesome Dave, and now is a great time to start expressin' your creativity, especially if your gunna keep buildin' your sexual energy. It's essential to have a direction and an outlet for it. One thing about energy is, it can either work with you or against you. It all depends on which way you want to focus it."

Bob began to unpack his books on the table. Some of them looked like they belonged inside an Egyptian pyramid. Dave was interested and came closer to inspect the treasure.

"I loved art and writing at school but I wasn't good enough to get into art at uni, so I've kind of just put it on the back burner."

"You really think that you're not good enough at it?" the Californian asked from behind a book.

"I dunno... I really enjoy it though," Dave replied.

"That's the thing with art," Bob continued. "Art is freedom and who doesn't enjoy freedom? As soon as rules or guidelines come in where creativity is involved, it suffocates the whole process. Go look at a five year old's painting and see the raw expression and freedom in it. It's so alive and real. When I was at high school, my music and art teachers all told me I was no good as well and it took me about ten years to find my creativity again after that. I really believed what they told me and I lost ten good years. Suppose that's why I'm so passionate about it now." He reached into the box with a big grin and pulled out a black sketch book. "Check these out!"

Dave sat down next to him as he flicked through dozens of masterpieces, from fine pencil portraits to striking, colourful, abstract pieces.

"They're brilliant! I had no idea I was in the company of Picasso!" he joked. Bob was deep in thought and barely even responded.

"You know Dave, what if our purpose here on earth was to be as joyful and creative as we could possibly be, each in our own unique way?" It kind of went over Dave's head and he sat there quietly with a puzzled look on his face. "What I'm trying to say is, that I feel very different to the majority of people on the planet. The majority seems to be living in the confines of society and their own conditionings and unfortunately there isn't a great deal of freedom in that."

Dave interrupted: "I think that's what happened to me with Grace. Each day I could feel a barrier come down that I didn't even know was there. It's helped me to see my limitations and the freedom that comes from that is epic. Lookin' back on my life, I can see how serious I was becomin'… and it was killin' me."

"Yeah man, that's what I'm talkin' about!" Bob said excitedly. "Imagine life was more about joy than seriousness… how would that be?"

Dave felt amazing just considering the possibilities. *Imagine never having to work at the hardware store again! Imagine how it would be to have a life filled with creativity and joy!* Dave had a vision of himself as a famous artist, standing in front of a huge, colourful painting of a dolphin. There were people from all walks of life gathered around bidding for the painting. $10,000… SOLD, he laughed to himself, realising it was more than possible.

"Gather some wood together Dave… we're having a beach fire ceremony tonight!" Bob sounded very official and Dave was caught a bit off-guard.

"What's the ceremony for?"

"Don't you worry 'bout that at this stage of the game dude. You'll find out soon enough," Bob said, still rolling with the policeman voice, which ended in laughter.

Dave knew not to pry any further and went to gather some wood. Another day was coming to a close and it was shaping up to be a breathtaking sunset. The clouds were set up perfectly and colours were already beginning to appear.

Far out, what a day! Dave bent down to stack

another piece of wood in his already loaded arms. He flashed on Grace and wondered how she was getting on. Any sadness he'd been carrying about her leaving was now gone and all that remained was a feeling of appreciation for all the experiences they'd shared and all she'd taught him. He was feeling much more comfortable with his sexual energy and also realised it was just the beginning into that area of exploration.

It was Dave's turn to cook and he created a delicious vegetable soup which included some homemade bread Pete had given him. Bob was quiet and didn't reveal an ounce of information about the ceremony. After dinner he disappeared into the Kombi and finally re-emerged carrying a small wooden box, a tanned leather pouch over his shoulder and a big jar full of strange looking liquid.

"Okay Dave, let's get this fire cranked up. Tonight is a very special night!" The two of them walked down onto the beach in front of the love shack. It was now dark and the sky was filled with luminous stars. The moon had not yet arrived, which just added juice to the brilliant star show. Dave was an expert in setting up fires and this one was no exception. Bob was acting a little weird; well, a little more so than usual. Ever since the idea of the ceremony had come up, he'd been very mysterious.

"So Dave, I feel you've come to a point in your life where you're at the crossroads... you feel ready to let go of the old and embrace the new. Your experience with that dolphin today was not just a coincidence. It was a blessing from Mother Nature and Great Spirit to usher you into a new stage of your life. All the early cultures worked with ceremony to anchor and celebrate these different stages. Tonight my friend, it's all about you!"

Bob opened up his small wooden box revealing some wrapped up herbs and a few colourful, sparkling crystals. From the pouch he took a piece of red material, a book and a bunch of various sized feathers strapped together at the base with leather.

"This looks exciting," Dave said nervously, giving an awkward little laugh. Bob laid the material down on the sand and proceeded to neatly arrange all his bits and pieces on top of it. Even the glass jar was placed there with precision. Out of the blue, came a BOOMING Californian voice:

"I light this fire to bring strength to this ceremony... to burn away the old and allow the new to rise up through the ashes." Bob struck a match and within seconds the fire was ablaze, throwing dancing sparks up into the night sky. "I call in the four directions!" He opened his arms widely, palms facing upwards. "I call in the warm air from the north... the expansive ocean to the west... I call in the east, place of the rising sun... and I call in the south, home of the almighty trees. I also call in the energies of Mother Earth and Great Spirit to be present with us tonight."

Dave was becoming concerned. He'd never heard anyone carry on like this before. He wondered who Great Spirit was. Either way, Bob was enjoying himself and Dave was bubbling with intrigue as to what may happen. Bob held the stick of herbs in the fire until one end was alight and took the feathers from the ground.

"This is white sage," he explained, "Native Americans use this as a ceremonial tool. The smoke is said to clear away old energies that are no longer serving you. Are you ready to let yours go?"

"Yes, I am super ready!" Dave responded passionately.

"Okay. Stand here facing the fire." Smoke was now billowing from the sage stick and Bob circled Dave, fanning it all around his body with the feathers. A bolt of electricity shot up Dave's back and he coughed loudly. "Obviously didn't need that one anymore!" Bob said with a laugh, beginning to lighten up a bit.

It was a magical process and Dave was definitely feeling something going on. Bob reached down and grabbed the book for the next stage of the event.

"After researching through many of the old texts, I have finally found a new name for you. This name will help you to remember who you really are. To embrace your joy, lightness and fun, your unlimited energy and creative potential. Your new name is... MAKARA!" Bob thundered, as though it was a grand finale circus act.

Some moments passed and Dave stood there a little uncertain. *A new name? Why do I need a new name?* he thought, confused.

"This means dolphin in an ancient Indian language," Bob continued, opening a thick, dirt brown coloured book. "I had no idea of the relevance this name has for you bro, but the more I researched it, the more it all became clear. This is sooooo you man! Here, check out these meanings." Bob turned a few more pages, found his notes and began to read them in the light of the now raging fire:

"There are three sounds that make up your new name. Ma, Ka and Ra. 'Ma' can be traced back to Hindu roots meaning 'birth mother' and also has ties in old Egypt with the 'goddess of truth and justice' named Maat. 'Ka' represents your spirit, your soul that you've carried for lifetimes, the guiding self you cannot see. 'Ra' through many cultures means sun and the radiant energy that brings life to our world." Bob paused and tended to the fire with a large stick, sending more sparkling orange ashes skyward.

Dave burst out laughing.

"You mean to say Dave's out the window and my new name is Makara! It sounds like an Indian curry or somethin'!" he exclaimed. Bob was a little taken back but realised his young friend didn't have the full understanding of what was he was on about.

"This whole re-naming ceremony is not somethin' that I've just made up man. In many old spiritual traditions, when a person was ready to let go of their old self, a new name was given. It's a way of startin' fresh, a way of re-birthing yourself almost, rememberin' who you truly are and givin' space for that to come forth. What happened to you today is a sure sign from nature, saying 'hey, you are ready'. And you are ready Dave. You wouldn't be here with me right now if you weren't."

"Fuck mate, I'm just not sure how down with it I

am. I know I really need to let go of my old, serious ways and start livin' with more joy and playfulness though... and it does sound like a strong name, but it's a little over the top, don't ya reckon!" Dave expressed reluctantly.

"Okay," Bob said, "let's do a little test then. I want you to stand here and say, 'my name is Makara' and see how it feels."

Dave stood up next to the red hot fire. He took a deep breath in and as he went to say it, the laughter came again. On his third attempt, he looked up to the night sky and yielded to the ceremony taking place. He spoke clearly and loudly with open arms: "MY NAME IS MAKARA!" A huge shooting star flew across the dark sky and burnt brightly all the way down to the horizon. Goose bumps sprung up all over his body. He felt very powerful. Bob quickly grabbed the glass jar.

"Okay, you need to drink this right now!" Bob said assertively, handing Makara the eccentric elixir he'd prepared earlier. Makara didn't think twice and gulped the whole contents down in one go. Coconut milk was definitely one of the ingredients but there was so much other stuff going on that his taste buds went into overdrive. Bob spoke up again:

"This magical potion will help anchor your new name and the joyful, playful, energised vibration that it carries."

Makara stood strong and silent next to the fire. He felt taller than before and his chest felt more open. A subtle shift had occurred and he was calm, happy and smiling on the inside. The fire crackled away and Bob slipped up to the love shack to get his drum, without Makara even knowing he'd left.

"The final part of the ceremony is all about celebration and gratitude!" Bob affirmed on his return, still breaking at the seams with enthusiasm. He began playing the drum and Makara's body started moving to the beat all by itself. The ocean, the rhythm, the fire and the starry night all set the stage for the ceremonial dance that was unfolding. Bob began picking up the pace and Makara responded with his movements, all the time staring intently into the fire. His dance was wild and free! The drums rang out across the bay and another shooting star exploded above them.

15. THE MIRROR

"Thanks for your help today Dave, I really appreciate it mate!" Pete said, sweat dripping from his forehead after a hard morning's work on the shovel.

"Yeah, no worries... but remember I told you I changed my name to Makara a few days ago," came the uneasy response.

"Oooh yeah, sorry mate," Pete replied, a touch embarrassed. "I'll do my best to remember next time."

Makara was beginning to question this whole name change thing. On the night, he'd eventually embraced his name and felt solid and grounded with it the next day. The last few days around camp however, had been a real challenge. People kept forgetting his new name and he was constantly explaining why he'd done it. He wasn't even sure himself any more.

The day after the ceremony, Makara had phoned his parents from Pete and Sally's house to let them know how he was and that he'd even changed his name. The excitement didn't last long though. His father had asked if he was taking drugs and his mother was very concerned and wanted to speak with Bob. Makara tried to explain why he'd done it and the significance, but it hadn't gone down too well at all. Dave's dad had even become quite upset, asking: "What's wrong with the name we gave you?"

Makara felt guilty and didn't know what to say. Luckily his phone card had ran out of credit. He was beginning to see clearly how letting go of his old self was going to be harder than he thought. He realised the changes were not only affecting him but also all of those around him. *How would it be to start totally fresh where no one knew me?* he pondered. *Even my parents aren't supporting me to live a more joyful, energised life. I don't get it!*

He walked slowly back to the love shack, breathing in the fresh morning air and enjoying the warmth of the sun. The desert offshore wind had been howling all night and today the ocean was dead flat.

"Aloha Makara!" came the warm greeting, as he approached the camp. "How's it all going man?"

"Yeah, aloha Bob," he replied, sounding a bit flat. "This whole name change thing is drivin' me up the wall. My parents think I'm off my head. The guy up there," pointing to the camp on the hill, "has decided to call me Mac and Pete keeps forgettin' it."

Bob came closer, looking straight into his eyes and spoke with clarity:

"Makara... you're birthing your new self and this is a very important time for you. There is a great lesson unfoldin' right now in all of this. What other people think of you is none of your business. If they don't get you or get your name, it doesn't matter. What matters is how you feel about yourself. You need to discover lovin' yourself first and stop lookin' outside for it. Lookin' on the outside will only bring you sufferin' man. If you truly want a more joyous life, self-love is the key."

Makara listened intently. The truth in Bob's words seemed to be going past his brain and hitting somewhere deeper.

"I get it... but how do I get more self-love?"

"You're already so on the right track dude. Everythin' Grace taught you about cultivatin' your energy through self-pleasurin' and honourin' yourself... that's a great start! Somethin' I learned which works well also is an exercise where you look into a mirror and tell yourself things like, 'you're a beautiful man, I love you, I appreciate you.' And it works really well. It's also much more challengin' than you think.

"We've all taken on so many conditionings and beliefs that we're ugly, unworthy, stupid or unlovable... and most of the time, we don't even know they're there. When you start lookin' in that mirror and appreciatin' yourself, your whole life begins to change. Imagine if everyone on the planet truly loved themselves! Do you think the world would be a better place?"

Makara walked over to Freedom and leaned in next to the side rear vision mirror to give it a go. Since they'd been on the road, he'd hardly looked at himself at all and it gave him a bit of a shock. His eyes did look bigger and they were more sparkly than he'd ever remembered. They'd possibly even changed colour? His hair was big, curly and messy and his face was brown and freckly. He was actually looking very alive and healthy.

"Hello," he said nervously to himself, looking deeply into his own eyes with the curiosity of a child.

Bob walked off into the shack to give him some space. Makara kept looking and no other words came. He knew the exercise and what he was meant to be doing, but nothing came and he began to get frustrated. All he could see was a young man who'd stuffed up in life, how he wasn't doing what everyone else was doing and how he felt he'd never amount to anything... ever! Makara kept looking until his eyes were so full of tears he couldn't see any more. He'd had enough and felt terrible. Only one thing could fix him now. He had to get into the ocean immediately to wash away the pain.

"Holy shit Bob... all I could say was 'hello' and now I feel awful," he said, passing through the love shack to get his towel.

"Don't worry man, it gets easier. Like anythin' it takes practice and the start is the toughest for sure. If you do a little bit everyday you'll be bouncin' around, all loved-up in no time!"

Today the water was crystal clear and extremely inviting. Makara dived in and instantly felt better. He wasn't sure why or how but no matter what was happening, the ocean always did the trick. He lay there floating on his back, drinking in the sunshine and letting his shoulders relax after the morning digging program. It was an awesome job he had with Pete, but some days it was bloody hard work.

They'd been digging out a few of the old toilet tanks, which were basically forty-four gallon drums sunk into the ground. By the time it came to dig them out they'd spent months composting, so it was more just like shovelling rich garden soil... thank God! Once that was all cleared out, the framework around the toilet was moved into the new position, ready for action. As there was no running water available, compost toilets were the best option and they worked well. They were quite cute actually. They had a rough little structure around them made out of timber and palm fronds for privacy. Some of the toilets had sensational views of the ocean and the point. You could even sit on the dunny and watch people surfing.

The camp was a friendly, small community of surfers, travellers and people from all over the world. Some people stayed for a few days whilst others pretty much lived there. Everyone had the same underlying reason that had drawn them there: to enjoy nature and slow life down. It was such a change having no electricity or fresh running water and Dave was learning a new appreciation for both. To organise dinner while it was still light and hit the hay as soon as it was dark had become the routine. Living simply and in tune with the natural rhythms of the day... what a way to live!

The days continued to slide by and Makara made an agreement with himself to practise his 'self-love' mirror exercise twice a day and as Bob had predicted, it was becoming easier. He'd also been experimenting with self-pleasuring when he had the space and was realising when he didn't ejaculate, his energy levels were phenomenal. Makara was also learning to enjoy his body more which was odd but also very liberating at the same time. He'd always focused on the negative aspects of his body and this was starting to change. It was such a relief to realise that he was actually a beautiful young man.

One particular morning, self-pleasuring went for well over half an hour and he managed to not 'let go'. That day he surfed for six hours straight and only came in 'cause he was starving. Overall, he was feeling awesome and wondered to himself why everyone didn't know this stuff? Guys always joked about 'wanking' and seemed to use it as a pressure release but Makara was learning there was far more to it than that.

After a few days of the ocean going flat again, the surf began to pump and a whole new bunch of campers arrived. There was a real buzz in the air and apparently a couple of days of epic surf were forecast. The first day wasn't all that it was cracked up to be, but the second day really turned on and after helping Pete out with the morning rounds, Makara wasted no time in getting out there. A perfectly lined-up four to six foot swell rolled into the bay, fanned by a light offshore breeze. Flawless conditions, with almost every wave offering a tube.

One of the new campers, this guy with a huge mop of bright red hair, was being a total wave pig and sending bad vibes through the whole crowd of surfers. He wanted every wave he could get his hands on and wasn't interested if it was someone else's turn. Makara waited patiently and eventually found himself on one of the best waves of the morning, that Pete had called him into. When Pete called you in, you knew it was yours!

Makara pulled straight into a huge pipe and was weaving his way through, when all of a sudden the red haired baboon decided to take off and 'drop in' on him. Makara yelled loudly but the guy went anyway, forcing him to straighten out in the tube to avoid a high speed collision. Red Mop didn't even make the take-off and they both got annihilated, coming up in the foam, with their legropes tangled and almost on top of each other. Makara's board was damaged and he was furious at this guy, calling him every name under the sun. Red Mop argued back and it almost came to blows, until the next wave hit them like a road-train, washing them both onto the razor sharp reef.

Makara returned back to the shack with cuts all over his feet, carrying a well and truly smashed-up board.

He was still fuming but the walk home had mellowed him out a lot.

"You should've seen this idiot drop in on me!" began Makara, as soon as he saw Bob. "It's one of those new roosters who arrived yesterday and he thinks he's the king of the point already. He even had a go at me for blowing up at him. The guy's an asshole. I don't even…"

Bob's hand shot up suddenly, making a stop sign in front of Dave's face. "Righto, ENOUGH!" he declared sternly. "I'm not going to stand here like a trash can for you to dump your anger into. Take it up the beach and give it to the sand! You know what to do."

Makara was not expecting this response from Bob at all and it made him even more enraged. The anger now bubbling ferociously and becoming extremely volcanic. He looked at Bob with a death stare, turned and took off down the beach as fast as his feet would carry him.

Why is Bob treatin' me like shit as well? What the fuck's goin' on? He began charging like a bull up the beach. He had so much energy and just kept running… his mind going a million miles per hour, reflecting on times in his life where he'd been unfairly treated. Tears came and went, and he just kept on running. Over the rocks, up onto the track and right out of the camp, oblivious of the cuts on his feet. Makara felt like he never wanted to see Bob again, or anyone at the camp for that matter. He began punching the air and screaming as he ran. He was beside himself with rage and just kept on running.

Eventually he stopped, well and truly exhausted, legs burning and feet aching. He leaned forward with his hands on his thighs, gasping for breath. He had just moved a mountain of anger and now in its place, was that newly familiar lake of calm. As his breath died down, he realised how quiet it was around him, almost too quiet. It looked as though the weather was turning and for the first day in weeks, the clouds were thickening up. There were only two options now: to keep walking away and spend a cold, hungry night alone in the desert or to head home.

On the long walk back, Makara was surprised at how far he'd actually gone. He was tired and thirsty. He gradually began to realise how much of an idiot he'd been abusing the guy in the surf and then proceeding to dump all his drama on Bob. It was very rare he became angry but when he did, he was almost out of control. The intensity was frightening. It was a part of him that he didn't like and tried to pretend it wasn't there a lot of the time, by being the peaceful, mister nice guy.

Even though his feet and body ached and he'd made a fool of himself earlier, he began to see the bigger picture. He saw and appreciated the strength in Bob's boundaries and once again, became aware of the free, amazing life he himself was living right now. He'd also had a bunch of great waves that morning before Red Mop had almost killed him! As Makara continued his walk home, waves of gratitude began washing over him.

He saw clearly how great all his life had been, especially when he focused on the positive aspects of each part. He even saw his parents in a whole new light and appreciated just how much they'd given over the years and also how much they loved him. He'd gone from one extreme to the other in a matter of hours and was now feeling so different. It was absurd how much was moving through him lately, how he was changing so much. It was like some deranged rollercoaster ride!

The sight of the camp ground brought a welcome relief. His thirst and hunger doubled in strength in the realisation that food and water were soon at hand. As he came up the beach towards the shack, Bob was outside packing up the cooker and all their gear was stacked against one of the outside walls.

"Aloha Bob. I'm really sorry for dumpin' all my crap on you earlier and I now appreciate the fact that you shut me down, so thank you." Bob stood up and moved towards him with open arms.

"I totally accept your apology bro." The two of them melted into a man hug, Makara relieved to be home.

"Mate... I also wanna say that I'm so grateful for everythin' you've done for me and all your support."

"Thanks for appreciatin' me man, that means a lot. It's been such an honour and a blessing to be part of your transformation. I've never seen anyone evolve so quickly and with so much courage before. I guess you were ready for it. Take today for example: you went from a ragin' bull to a buddha in one afternoon. Some people carry anger like that for weeks, years even. It's awesome what you're doin' dude! On another note, I've decided to pack her up. Apparently there are four or five days of rain and onshores comin', so it's a good time to peel out."

"Sounds good... Sorry I wasn't here to help you pack," Makara said, feeling a little shaken by the news and grabbing a bottle of water for a well needed drink.

"It's all good man. I've actually been enjoyin' the process of tidying up. We've had a good run here and I'm feelin' ready for a change of scene ya know."

Dave had another big drink and leaned up against the shack to asses the cuts on his feet that were now really starting to hurt. Bob came closer to check them out.

"You've done a good job on those dude, that reef is so unforgivin' hey. You get any urchin spines in there?" he asked, pulling a chair over for Makara to sit on.

"I dunno, haven't had a good look yet."

"I'll grab some water and we'll get these feet cleaned up," Bob said, snapping into action. "You don't wanna treat reef cuts lightly man. I've learned that lesson a few times already."

Bob had all the cuts on both feet cleaned up and dressed in no time. He had his own 'Bob style' First Aid Kit which contained all the usual dressings and band aids but there was his own natural twist on things too. He used tea tree oil for disinfecting the cuts and was even carrying homeopathic remedies to help with healing and boosting the immune system. He had Makara put a bunch of tiny, white, sweet tasting balls under his tongue and explained briefly to him how they worked. Most of it was a bit hard to grasp but he got the overall picture that they'd be helping.

Bob packed his kit up and headed for the van. Half way over he turned back to Makara. "Also, before I forget... while we're on the subject of appreciation and gratitude, I've got another great little exercise to add to your bag of tricks. You can even use the book Denise gave you for it. The idea is, before you go to bed each night, list down twenty things in your life that you're grateful for. Remember, one of those CD's we were listenin' to spoke about it. I think she was talking about doin' five things, but twenty before bed is next level. It's powerful and really gets you focusin' on the bright side of life. We all have so much more to be grateful for and appreciate than we even know. So often we overlook the basics; access to fresh drinking water, a warm bed to sleep in, or just walkin' around in theses healthy bodies... Y'know what I'm sayin'?"

"Wow Bob, sounds great! I'll start tonight. On my walk back today, I actually saw how I'd been overlookin' so many amazin' aspects of my life. I wonder why we always get caught up focusin' on the negatives?"

"I often wonder the same thing myself. It's like the ego just loves to juice negativity, 'cause without it, it can't survive. It thrives on the stuff! The human mind can be such a monkey sometimes," Bob replied, rolling his eyes. "Though once we get into that state of constant gratitude and appreciation, our whole world transforms before our eyes. It's funny 'cause we generally don't even have to change anythin' outside of us, all we need to change is the way we see things. Seems so simple doesn't it."

Makara downed some more water, had an emergency sandwich and helped Bob pack up the camp. They were ready to roll in no time. It was a shock to be leaving so quickly and Makara had no idea what the next stop would be. It'd been a crazy day and the idea of moving on brought some relief... plus his board was now unrideable after its meeting with the rocks.

On the way out, they dropped in to see Pete and Sally for a cuppa. Pete was bummed to be losing his number one assistant and thanked Makara, by his new name this time, for all his hard work.

"It's been my pleasure Pete. I'm really grateful for the experience and spendin' time with ya. I've learned a lot... especially about tube ridin'!" he finished, filling the office with laughter. "Nah, seriously though," he continued jokingly, "this place has truly changed my life... I've even ended up with a new name!"

The afternoon was getting on and Bob wanted to get the dirt track out of the way before dark and potential rain. "Thank you so much Pete and Sally, for everything," he said, giving them a big hug with his long, matted hair going everywhere. Bob was looking wilder and wilder as the adventure progressed, to the point where he was now on the verge of the complete 'homeless bum' look. If you'd never met him before he'd be quite a scary proposition.

Bob pulled Freedom over at the top of the hill overlooking the camp and jumped out, Makara following suit. "Okay little bro," he said excitedly, rubbing his hands together. "We may as well keep rollin' with the gratitude vibration. How 'bout we choose five things each that we've appreciated over the last few weeks here and say them out loud. Kinda like a farewell ceremony. I'll begin."

He spread his feet about hip-width, closed his eyes and took a couple of deep breaths.

"I am grateful for this life-givin', magical ocean, which has fed us, cleaned us, given us swells to ride and even washed our pots. I am grateful for the sunshine and the perfect weather we've had. I am extremely grateful we got to stay in the love shack. I am grateful for the new friends I've made and I'm grateful that my trusty van is runnin' so well."

Bob paused for a moment and then stretched his arms out to the sides, raised them up above his head with the palms facing each other. He then, ever so slowly, brought them down into a prayer position in front of his heart. "Thank you, thank you, thank you... I also give thanks to this ancient land and honour the original inhabitants and the ancestors that came before me."

As he finished speaking, a flock of twenty or thirty black cockatoos came from nowhere and flew overhead, their Jurassic screeches sending shivers down Makara's spine. It was the first time he'd seen so many together, their red, striped tail feathers throwing bright colour into the clouded afternoon sky.

"WOW! The power of gratitude!" Makara said, bewildered by what had just happened. "Okay, I'll have a go now but I very much doubt I can top that. I'm grateful for the epic waves we got to ride. I'm really grateful for my time with Grace who schooled me in things I'd never imagined. I'm grateful for getting a job to offset my rent durin' our stay. I'm very grateful to you Bob, for bringin' me to this amazin' place... and I'm grateful for my new name and the unlimited possibilities that lay before me!" he finished, inspired and full of energy.

They both stood there looking back over the camp and the ocean in silence. To the north over the sea, it was already raining. Suddenly, the sun decided to burst through a hole in the clouds and completely light up the sky. A luminous, half rainbow appeared, unfolding right before their eyes. Makara began laughing:

"I didn't think I could pull it off but I'm gettin' the feelin' a burst of sun and a kick ass rainbow might be better than a bunch of birds! What do ya reckon Bob?"

"Yeah... I was pretty impressed with mine, but man... you seem to have stolen the show," his companion said, throwing his arms into the air to appreciate the spectacular sight before them. The rainbow was now a full arc of vivid colour, bridging the sea and land. Bob looked at Makara with a smile: "The power of appreciation, hey!"

16. FOLLOW THE RAINBOW

"This is no place to camp ya stinkin hippies!" came a loud, stern voice, followed by a car door slamming shut. The lads had arrived to town quite late the previous night and set up camp in the supermarket car park to keep it simple. Apparently some of the locals didn't take kindly to it which bought a few giggles from inside the van. They must have slept in 'cause outside was already a buzz with trolleys, shoppers and cars. It was the closest they'd been to a huge selection of food in weeks, so no time was wasted in getting inside the shop.

"How's the smell in this aisle?" Makara said, trying to hold his breath as they passed all the cleaning products and laundry liquids.

"Yeah, it's the off gas... toxic huh," Bob stated, like

he knew what he was talking about. After sucking in fresh air for weeks, the supermarket was like being on another planet. They both held onto the trolley and sailed down the aisle as though it was a big skateboard.

"Do you eat these?" Makara asked, holding up a packet of corn chips, thinking they'd be a good, healthy option.

"Maybe... what's the ingredients?" Bob asked suspiciously.

Makara turned the packet over searching diligently. "Okay, we've got corn, canola oil, sugar, flavouring number 113/ 234 and preservative 202."

Seeing the sugar, the numbers and the preservatives, he placed the package back on the shelf. Shopping with Bob was always an adventure 'cause he read the ingredients on everything and there was no way in the world he was eating 'numbers'. If it wasn't natural and good for his body, it wasn't going into his mouth. Apart from his rough looks, he was a shining example of energy and health, so Makara figured he must be doing something right.

They'd almost run completely out of tucker and a big shop was in order. It was bizarre to have everything available at your fingertips after weeks of just living off what they had. In the last few days at the love shack, the food had run down so much they'd gotten extra creative with their meals. Makara had even come up with a baked bean and oat creation that was very interesting!

The checkouts were busy and Bob spotted a

winner with an old lady who had almost finished.

"Go for that one," he pointed to Makara, enjoying the game. "I just need to go and grab somethin' I forgot."

Makara began stacking the produce onto the counter, imagining the tasty meals they'd be creating. The little old lady in front of him went to pay and after she'd emptied the entire contents of her hundred year old looking purse, she came up $2.60 short. She went into a mild panic, apologising and rustling through her shopping to see which item she would have to go without. Before she even had a chance to find one, Makara spoke up:

"I'm more than happy to help you out," he said, reaching into his pocket and pulling out a bunch of change. "Here's $2.60 right here," and handed it to the overweight, checkout-chick who seemed very surprised.

The old lady approached Makara and shook his hand. She was stronger than she looked!

"I didn't think that sort of thing happened any more," she said, gratefully looking up at him.

"Well…it's just started to change and it's happenin' again!" he replied confidently.

The little old lady continued looking at him and a big smile came across her face. "That's great. The world will be a better place for it," she said warmly, with a twinkle in her eye.

By now, Bob had returned with his new toothbrush and wondered what all the fuss was about. The old lady grabbed her bags and turned once more to acknowledge Makara's generosity: "Thanks again young man!" and she walked off, her smile now even bigger than before.

The goods were now being scanned and the checkout chick spoke up: "I've been working here for a year and a half and it's the first time I've ever seen that sort of generosity... well done mate! If I were you I'd go next door and buy a lotto ticket. I believe you've got some good karma coming your way."

Makara had no idea what 'karma' was but one thing was for sure, he was feeling great and loved the idea of getting a lotto ticket. "Thanks, I might just do that," he said, stacking things into a green, material bag. *It's amazing how something so small could have such a big effect, he thought to himself. Only $2.60 to get a grandma smiling and some good karma... whatever that is.*

He filled Bob in on the details, who was proud of his young apprentice and confirmed the sort of positive ripple effect spontaneous actions like that can create. Makara wasted no time and went straight outside and into the Newsagent next door.

"I'd like to buy a lotto ticket please!" he announced excitedly to the man behind the counter, who looked a little confused.

"Right... we've got loads to choose from, what sort are you after?" As he was speaking, Makara looked down and beneath the glass bench top saw the selection of sparkling Scratchies. One, which immediately caught his eye, had a huge, colourful rainbow landing in a pot of gold and WIN UP TO $10,000 written across the rainbow. He knew that was the one.

"I'd love that colourful rainbow Scratchie thank you," he said assertively.

The man tore it off and put it in a little paper bag. Makara paid and was out the door like lightning to find Bob and share the fun. The two of them sat down on a bench under a tree and Makara began scratching intently. Half way through game four, the second last game, $3,000 came up twice and there were two more pots of gold to scratch. *Just imagine what $3,000 right now could do?* he thought, as all the possibilities flooded through his mind.

"YEESSSSSSSSSSSSSS!!!!" Makara screamed. He stood up and threw his right hand into the air, holding the Scratchie tightly in his left. He'd just won $3,000 and was absolutely beside himself. "YEEESSSSSSS!! I'VE DONE IT!!!"

By now, Bob was jumping up and down as well, after initially being frozen as he witnessed the last pot of gold in the row reveal another $3,000. Makara was ecstatic. People leaving the supermarket were a little suspicious of the two hippies jumping around and were taking a wide berth around them with their trolleys.

Makara walked straight back into the Newsagent to claim his prize. Luckily it was the owner serving and he knew exactly how to handle a winning ticket. He was super happy as well! He did all the official checks and within five minutes, placed a huge stack of $50 notes on the counter. Makara received it gratefully and counted the notes out one by one to check that it was all there. He'd occasionally handled big amounts of money at the hardware store but this was his and it was different. As he bunched the notes together and tucked them into the zipper pocket in his shorts, he felt a huge weight lift off his shoulders. He thanked the owner a hundred times and ran back out to celebrate more with Bob, who had a massive smile from ear to ear.

"Lunch is on me!" he yelled, slapping his pocket full of money and laughing in total disbelief at what had just happened.

Bob got up and gave him a big hug, saying with encouragement: "Well done bro... See what happens when you shine your light."

"I never thought it could be this easy," Makara said, with tears welling up in his eyes. "I feel so looked after." Bob held him tight, reassuring him and explaining that this was still just the beginning.

Pete and Sally had told them about a fantastic new health food shop in town that was worth checking out. Apparently they did lunches, juices and a vast selection of other good stuff. Once the shopping was packed into Freedom, they went on the hunt for the health store. Being a smallish town, it didn't take them long to find. Pete and Sally had been right on the money: the place was really well done, it was huge! Half of it was a conventional health food shop and the other half was set up as a groovy looking restaurant with indoor plants, comfy couches and rustic timber tables... it even had a water feature inside!

The lads were famished and grabbed a table to assess the menu. This was definitely Bob's kind of establishment with just about everything on the menu being fresh, local and organic. The 'Superfood Lunch Combo' jumped out at them and it consisted of a tempeh burger with salad and a superfood, green smoothie that had almost half a page of ingredients in it. The waitress was friendly and reassured them it was a wise choice. Once again they were living the dream.

Makara looked across at Bob and asked inquisitively:

"So what actually is 'karma'?"

"It's pretty simple man. The way I understand it is, if you do somethin' good, good things show up for you and if you do somethin' bad... well, you get the picture. And what just happened for you was the most instant good karma I've ever seen!" Bob laughed, still totally blown out that Makara had just won three grand.

"Yeah, I get it. I didn't realise it was that simple. When I was younger, I had a classic example of that but the other way around. I helped some mates break into a car which was fun at the time but obviously not a really cool thing to do. The following day my two week old skateboard was stolen from outside the movie store. I guess this karma stuff works pretty quickly for me."

"That's exactly it dude," Bob said, pouring himself a glass of bottled spring water. "One of my teachers passed on a healthy rule of thumb to live by and that is to treat others the way you want to be treated.

Again, it's so simple and a great one to remember."

The beautiful waitress returned with a large smile and two plates brimming with colour and life.

"Here are your burgers guys and it's your lucky day, as Rhonda was baking this morning: you've got homemade spelt bread," she said very proudly.

Makara smiled back at her: "You're definitely right there... it is our lucky day!" which brought a laugh from Bob.

The food was delicious and in a way the salad was similar to Bob's style of creation: so much variety, taste and juiciness. Once they were consumed, the green smoothies arrived and holy moly, they were out of control! It was another main course in itself and they decided to have a look around the store to let the burgers digest a bit before hooking into the smoothies.

Makara was drawn to a large notice board on the wall loaded with various flyers and adverts. Things for sale, people wanting to car pool and then something caught his eye: a brightly coloured big sign with a rainbow across the middle of it, advertising a 'conscious living festival'. It described an event which was drug and alcohol free with a focus on celebrating life through music, dance, yoga, meditation and creative workshops. The best thing was that it started in two days' time. The hair on Makara's arms stood up and a feeling of expansion grew in his heart. He glanced around, seeing Bob researching packets of dry seaweed in one of the aisles.

"Bob, come and check this out!" he said loudly, to

get his attention. Bob wasted no time after hearing the aliveness in his voice. "Do you know how far this place is from here?" Makara said, pointing to the funny-sounding name of the town.

"It'd have to be about a three hour drive I reckon. I've heard of this festival before, but never been. Apparently it's awesome."

Makara smiled confidently, realising they had money, time and no set plans for anything else. "Wow Bob, I hadn't even thought about where we were off to next, but I think I've found our new destination."

"I'm in for sure," Bob replied, rubbing his hands together, "This festival has been on my list of things to do for a few years now."

They both stood there soaking up all the info from the flyer and borrowed a pen and paper from the waitress to jot down some details. There was even the option for guests to arrive a few days early to settle in and enjoy the place. It was a plan and they decided to hit the road after getting a few more supplies and enjoying their smoothies, which were easily the best ever!

The forecast rain still hadn't arrived and the sun was shining. Once on the road, Makara shared with Bob how he was puzzled by the way everything was flowing so easily. He'd totally forgotten about his money worries at the desert surf camp and up until an hour ago, didn't even know where they were going next, but was relaxed about it at the same time. Bob hammered the point home about gratitude and appreciating your life.

"Once you begin to change your vibration from fear to trust and positivity, miracles start to happen. It's actually an ancient spiritual law that states, 'when you are grateful for what you do have, more good will show up in your life'. Your previous concerns about not havin' enough money created more of not havin' enough money. Now you're replacin' fear with appreciation and look what's happenin'!" Bob looked across, filled with joy and Makara nodded his head.

"It's awesome isn't it!"

The whole picture was slowly sinking in for Makara and he was starting to get it. *If it was really this easy, why wasn't everyone doing it?* he thought. He'd never looked at life and money like this before and it was as if you had to look at it upside down or back to front or something. He thought of two of his friends who'd already bought houses and had to come up with hundreds and hundreds of dollars every week for the next thirty years and one of them didn't even like his job. He wondered how many other people would be in similar situations and if they took the time to appreciate their lives. He mentioned his friends situation to Bob.

"Yeah, that can definitely be a nasty trap and it's a bit of a modern human dilemma in the west..."

"In the west??" Makara interrupted.

"Yeah, the 'west' is like the modern industrialised world of Europe, America and Australia. Even though the 'east' is quickly becoming similar, in countries such as India, a lot of the population are just happy to get some food and shelter each day. Man... we seem to get so caught up in havin' the biggest house, biggest TV and shiniest car that we become slaves to the system. We end up like stressed out robots rather than the free, creative, fun loving beings we were put here to be."

He reached down to change the music. The town was now far behind and the country they were travelling through was different. There were hills and mountains appearing and it was much greener than on the coast.

"A few years back, I ended up with this horror credit card debt and that taught me a very good lesson. I was payin' hundreds of dollars per month in interest to the bank. It was nuts! Eventually I got it sorted and I clearly remember the day when I cut my cards up. It was extremely liberatin' and one of the best things I've done. That credit card is another nasty little trap if used unwisely. I now prefer the old fashioned method of 'if you ain't got it don't spend it' and that seems to be workin' well. And then, if you really want somethin', you gotta get creative and make it happen man. That's super empowerin' and can be loads of fun too!" Bob looked across at Makara briefly: "Like you with the buskin' idea and workin' with Pete and winnin' that money!!"

He paused and laughed, still flabbergasted by the day's proceedings. Makara joined in the laughter and spoke up loudly over the noise of the Kombi and the music, to let his excitement out: "Imagine if life could always be this easy and fun!"

The afternoon drive was filled with positive

vibrations, enthusiasm, and a fresh perspective on life. For Makara, it was always radically expanding to spend time with Bob, a real education. He realised he hadn't gained entrance into the university of his choice but he'd ended up in a different kind of school. It was the school of life and adventure, and he was loving every minute of it.

The time flew by and suddenly they were only ten kilometres from their destination. Signs for the festival with arrows and balloons were already starting to appear, so they knew they were on the right track. The steep mountains they'd come over had now been reduced to rolling green hills with rivers and trees. It was breathtaking country.

You couldn't miss the entry. They'd created a huge rainbow arch that you drove under to enter. It was a real work of art and Bob pulled up directly underneath it to take a photo.

"Jump up on the roof Makara, and throw your arms in the air. We can't miss this opportunity." Makara slipped out the window and climbed easily up onto the roof. He threw his arms up, much to the delight of Bob, who was laughing and racing around capturing all the angles. They hadn't even passed the front gate and were already having a ball. It was a good sign of what lay ahead.

Another couple of cars rolled up and the lads promptly brought the photo-shoot to a close as Freedom was blocking the entrance. On they drove and the two of them were like kids in a toy store.

Check this out! Check that out! There was lots to take in; fruit trees everywhere, cute, earthy-looking Eco bungalows dotted about, veggie gardens full of colour and creativity, people and kids of all shapes and sizes. The festival hadn't officially started as yet but there was definitely something going on here.

They followed the signs to the camping area, which was magnificent as well. It consisted of a huge, flat, fairly open space with the odd tree and it backed onto a winding river which looked excellent for swimming. Bob found a perfect spot next to a few old trees to park and pointed out a good place to set up the tent.

"We'll set the tent up over there man, then we've both got our own space and I won't be woken up in the mornin' with your heavy breathin' and self-pleasurin' exercises!" he laughed.

"Sounds perfect!" Makara replied, joining in the laughter and jumping out of the van to assess his new campsite.

They agreed to set up first and then go check the place out. The dome tent was erected without much fuss and it was a beauty. Once inside, it was huge and Makara could almost stand bolt upright in the centre. He loved sleeping in tents; the fresh air, the rustle of the wind on the canvas. The bed and sleeping bag went in and he then rounded up all his possessions which comprised of one backpack! And he was sorted.

One last thing he had to take care of was his pocket full of cash. He quizzed Bob about it and they decided to stash it in a secret compartment at the back of a drawer in the van. It was the ultimate spot. For Makara, it felt great to handle the big wad of money again and he spoke up confidently, "I am soooooo grateful for winning this! Thank you, thank you, thank you!!"

17. LOVE CELEBRATION

"Another two beautiful men have arrived!" came the clear vibrant voice, of a short grey-haired man, walking towards Bob and Makara. "Welcome. My name is Swami," he said, throwing his arm's wide open to whoever wanted to receive the first hug. Bob jumped in, totally consuming the tiny old man with his long, wiry frame and that awesome mop of hair.

"Aloha! Bob is my name."

"Well, aloha to you too Bob. I'm so happy that you're both here. We're in for a special week!" Swami moved towards Makara and gave him a big welcome hug.

"Hey Swami, my name is Makara."

"Aloha Makara. Aloha, that's cool... I haven't heard that one for years," he said, chuckling to himself. "The day is getting on and I would love to show you guys around before night comes. You're going to get the 'extra special sunset tour'... how does that sound?"

"We'd love that," Bob said, grateful for their warm reception.

Swami was 65 years of age and had been at the community for near on thirty years. He and a dozen of his friends had come together to create a different way of living and by the looks of things, they'd done a very good job. Swami's body was ageing but the shine in his eyes and his enthusiasm for life was inspiring, he seemed to carry this childlike innocence with him and his total lack of seriousness was right up the lads' alley. Already the laughter had begun!

They followed him along a winding path through the trees which led to this huge, funky building. It was simple and earthy on the outside and once inside, they were greeted by an explosion of bright colours and a well organised space.

"So, first things first. Welcome to 'The Happy Belly', our famous eating area. We are expecting hundreds of people for the festival and when it's in full swing, this kitchen over here will be all hands on deck. Tonight there will be a basic meal if required. And tomorrow... well, tomorrow night they'll be packed in here like sardines!"

After weaving their way through some more garden paths and past a life size Buddha sculpture, they arrived at another big building of similar appearance to the last one. It was all so neat and well looked after, Makara was impressed.

"This is our Meditation and Celebration Hall," Swami announced proudly. "Living in a community isn't all as romantic as it appears to be, and over the years this hall has been our saviour. One of the keys to making a community work is for the people living together to share a similar vision. Our vision here has primarily been based on growing in consciousness through meditation and opening our hearts. We honour ourselves, each other, Mother Earth and celebrate our amazing lives in every moment... well, when we remember!" Swami took a deep breath, looked out towards the last rays of sunset and relaxed against the rail at the base of the stairs.

"You know, we're all human and when we live side by side and spend a lot of time together, stuff comes up. It's natural, we've all had different computer programmers... I mean different parents," he laughed. "We all see the world differently so our commitment here over the years has focused on being as open and honest as possible in every situation, and slowly but surely the ego just falls away. I wouldn't change the way I live for anything in the world. I spent the first half of my life in an isolated, suburban brick box surrounded by fences, and sure it did the job for a while, but once you get a taste of community life with its richness and connection, there is no turning back."

Swami really loves a chat, thought Makara, realising the sunset tour was more of a Swami talking tour and in fact it was almost dark already.

"Let's go in," Swami continued with excitement, springing up the stairs like a six year old. There was a cute sign at the door which read, LEAVE YOUR MIND AND YOUR SHOES AT THE DOOR. Makara followed the directions and as he stepped into the hall, his whole body went to goose bumps and he felt an overwhelming urge to giggle.

"The energy's great in here, isn't it!" Swami reflected, as if knowing what had just happened. There were a dozen people inside cleaning up and organising the space. They barely even noticed the three of them enter the hall.

"What an awesome space," Bob added, surveying the whole room. The way they'd built the roof gave it the feeling of being inside a pyramid. Across the timber floor to the other side of the room, revealed two thumping big speakers and an area where live music would be performed. Just being in there made Makara feel like dancing!

Swami finished the tour by taking them to the information hut. Each day of the festival, the schedule of workshops and events would go up on the noticeboard there. If you had any questions about anything, this was the place to ask. Night had now fully arrived.

"That's enough for today," Swami said, completing his tour and sharing a few goodbye hugs.

"Thank you so much for your welcome tour, Swami, we appreciate it very much," Bob said, putting his hand over his heart.

"My pleasure. You guys are going to have so much fun here, I just know it."

Swami disappeared up one of the paths and the two of them eventually found their way back to the campsite. Bob knocked up a simple, healthy dinner of 'nori rolls' in the van and it was an early night to bed. Makara sat in his tent with a little light and wrote twenty things he was grateful for that day. Wow! There were so many, he actually ended up with forty! *This was easily the best day ever*, he thought to himself, drifting off to sleep.

By midday the next day, the campsite was almost full and the whole place was buzzing. Cars, tents, caravans, buses, you name it, they were all rolling in, one after the other and finding their camp-sites for the next week. Makara went off by himself to explore the rest of the magical property. Swami's tour the previous night had barely scratched the surface. He found two inviting swimming holes that even had their own little beach. Of course he found the fruit trees and even sampled some of the produce.

Makara was very happy he'd already passed level one and level two of 'Hug Training' because they were coming at him from every angle. He was now much more relaxed with hugs and thoroughly enjoying them, even with the men. To introduce himself as Makara and only have positive response, was a real breath of fresh air as well. With brand new friends there were no judgments or fears, plus many people he met had unusual names as well, with a variety of different meanings. Makara took great joy in sharing the story behind his name and everyone was genuinely interested.

The following day at sunrise was the Opening Ceremony of the festival. Makara had set his alarm and woken early to do some self-pleasuring and raise his energy beforehand. He was elated to have his own space again and was starting to get the hang of drawing sexual energy up his spine. *What a delicious way to start the day*, he thought, moaning to himself and enjoying his own energy. Makara was feeling fantastic and ready for the day. It was a clear, crisp morning and soon everyone would be meeting on the huge grass area next to the Meditation Hall.

He rounded up Bob and they made for the oval. On the way there, a group of four gorgeous young women came past them, skipping, singing and holding hands. Makara lit up and couldn't resist the opportunity. He grabbed hold of Bob's hand and started skipping after them in hot pursuit. Once the girls realised they were being chased, they picked up the pace and began giggling a lot. Each time the all-male skipping team almost caught them, the laughter went to the next level. It was out of control and the perfect alarm clock for all the campers that were still asleep. They arrived in stitches, puffing, panting, and now all wide awake.

The sun still wasn't up yet and that beautiful pre-dawn bluey, purple-colour filled the sky. There was already a large crowd of people gathered; some silent, some talking, some stretching and some looking like they were still sleeping. On the verandah of the Meditation Hall, Makara spotted a band setting up, complete with drum kit and a bunch of other instruments that he couldn't quite see from where he was.

People kept arriving till the huge grass space didn't look so huge anymore and then the music began. It started with a soft, slow guitar that gently woke those that were still half asleep. The rhythm increased, other instruments chimed in and soon the whole oval was a vibrant sea of dancing bodies. This was extreme next level for Makara. A couple of hundred people dancing at sunrise for no real reason in particular other than 'celebrating our amazing lives', as Swami had put it.

Makara was quite self-conscious at first, and as he began to look around, he realised there was no right or wrong way to dance and totally loosened up. There were kids running around, old people swaying like trees, one woman was going absolutely wild and no one seemed to care what anyone else was doing. The sun began to rise, throwing brilliant colours across the sky and the music was pumping! Bob was next to Makara and his big hair was going everywhere with his erratic moves.

After a couple of long songs, the music slowed, eventually stopping. A sweet woman's voice drifted out across the masses of content, smiling faces.

"Good morning beautiful people. Thank you all so much for showing up here today and bringing with you so much love and freedom. Welcome," she said, looking around at everyone. "I honour and give thanks to 'the native people of this ancient land', and to the ancestors that have come before us… I call in their blessings for this festival."

She then gave clear instructions for everyone to join hands in one big circle. It seemed like an impossibility due to so many people but within a minute or so, the circle was formed. Makara had lost Bob altogether and had two complete strangers on either side of him but they didn't feel like strangers at all. The feeling he had in his heart, standing there in that immense circle of people was almost overwhelming. He looked around at all the delighted faces, shining in the morning light and was so grateful to be where he was, right at that moment!

"What a blessing for humanity this is!" came the voice over the microphone again. "Here we are, over two hundred people from all parts of the globe, from all walks of life, gathered here this morning in peace, love and celebration. We will stand here in silence for the next five minutes and during that time, please hold an intention to send this love and this joy out into the world, especially for those that are needing it... and do not forget our true Mother, the earth beneath our feet. She needs your love and healing now more than ever before. This festival is officially open and I hope you all have a fun and enlightening week. Thank you, namaste, enjoy the silence."

For about thirty seconds you could've heard a pin drop. It was kind of eerie, so quiet... then a restless baby cried out breaking the silence, then it was quiet again. Makara focused on sending out love to his family and friends and his heart continued to expand. He wondered how they were all going and a little smile came to his face when he thought, *if only they could see me now!*

Five minutes flew by... and then the silence was ended by that same beautiful guitar. The sunrise celebration and dance fiesta continued. Makara was feeling phenomenal; so open, so free and his dance was beginning to reflect that. He himself was now getting wild and crazy, having an absolute blast.

At one stage he looked up and right there in front of him was the most stunning young woman he'd ever seen. The way she moved her body, the way her long, brown hair danced across her shoulders... it was love at first sight. Makara tried to not look too much and freak her out, but it was tough. The music continued and had now transformed into some funky, gypsy rhythm that the crowd was loving. She moved closer to Makara and when they both looked up to avoid bumping into each other, their eyes met.

Her face was magnificent; brown, soft-looking skin with these big, honey-coloured eyes that shot right through him. She returned his smile and electricity exploded through his entire body. The music kept pumping and the brown haired goddess disappeared back into the crowd. Makara continued the dance, feeling now even more alive, with a new vision of beauty etched into his mind.

Eventually he was exhausted and breakfast was calling. This dancing thing was a different kind of fitness to surfing and his legs were burning. He passed by the info hut and grabbed a program on his way back to camp. He had a poem brewing and pulled out his writing book once back in the tent.

There She Is
WOW! There she is,
Such sweetness, such joy, such aliveness.
My heart dances and stops at once.
There is fear, excitement and fun all together.
The morning sun lights up her face,
A smile so simple and real.
An energy like a light, rainbow rain.
We are so blessed to dance together.
All of us, here in the bliss.
Gratitude roars from my heart.
A waterfall rushes from my being.
Do I need to do anything?
Do I need to be anyone?
It is, as it is, as it is....
Already more than enough.

Bob eventually got back and they shared their standard muesli breakfast and debriefed about the morning. Bob was looking so good and reckoned he was glowing from the inside out with love. He declared that being in that space with so many others was one of the biggest joys of being human. Makara agreed and explained his experience of connecting with a gorgeous young woman during the dance.

They studied the program for the day which was offering everything under the sun. You could do Yoga, Tai Chi, Meditation, a Singing and Acting workshop, Heart Circle and even something called Laughing Buddha... and that wasn't even half of what was available! Bob was hanging out for some Tai Chi and Makara was drawn to the laughing Buddha, even though he didn't know what it was.

"Enjoy your Tai Chi bro," he said, before cruising off to find his workshop.

"Thanks man... enjoy the ride," Bob replied, half way through brushing his teeth.

A group of about thirty people were gathered on a nice grass area near the river. The facilitator was dressed like a human banana, which already had the laughter flowing. He was a big, fattish man with red cheeks and a beard.

Looks a bit like Father Christmas or that drunk guy Charley from the caravan park, Makara thought. The Big Banana explained the rules and how it all worked. You weren't even allowed to speak but could use 'gibberish' or nonsense language only.

The first exercise was to go around the circle and introduce yourself in this nonsense language and then actually say your name at the end. Makara was so focused on the Big Banana, he hadn't even noticed the woman from the dance that morning who was only three places to his right. When it was her turn she did a cute little dance and made a few noises, followed by 'Citrine' in a strange accent. Makara was in love already but now he was also intrigued.

The workshop was hilarious. You got to act like animals and do all sorts of fun, little improvised performances. It was like being a kid again and the Big Banana had such a deep, loud belly laugh that once he got going, it triggered the whole group. Makara got to pair up with Citrine during one exercise in which they had to act as if they'd been out drinking all night and they were stumbling home together. Makara had a pretty well rehearsed routine and by the looks of it, Citrine did too!

Once it finished, Makara got stuck chatting with this guy from Japan who was very friendly, but all he really wanted to do was to meet Citrine. He missed his opportunity though, as she had walked off with a guy. *So perhaps she has a boyfriend*, he thought, a little bummed. Either way, there was just something about her and he had a burning desire to find out what it was.

Two days passed and the festival was now in full swing. It was by far the best thing Makara had ever experienced and he was constantly meeting interesting people from all over the world. The hugs continued, he'd never danced so much in all his life, the celebration, the joy... love was in the air! For two whole days he hadn't even spotted Citrine once and was beginning to think she'd left.

For the last two days, Makara had been doing this wild, early morning, Active Meditation which involved chaotic breathing, emotional release and jumping up and down like a Zulu warrior. It was radical, but it left him feeling clear, peaceful and energised... he loved it. He'd heard they were creating delicious juices for breakfast at The Happy Belly and on the third morning it was all he could think about in the last stage of the Meditation.

It was still early and there weren't many people around. He ordered a large Super Zinger Juice and they knocked it out for him on the spot. He headed for some tables which were outside in the morning sun. As he stepped out the door, his heart stopped as he saw Citrine sitting alone in the sunshine having a juice. The morning Meditation was having a profound impact on Makara and instead of freezing or shrinking away, he walked straight up to the table, feeling fairly relaxed and somewhat confident.

"Aloha, do you mind if I join you?" he asked, a part of him unable to believe what he was actually doing.

"Yes, good morning, please sit down," Citrine replied in her broken English, with a strong, sexy accent that Makara guessed was French.

"My name is Makara," he said, putting out his hand across the table, still way too nervous to jump straight into a hug.

"I am Citrine," she replied, pushing out her chair, standing up and leaning over the table. She took his hand, pulled herself towards him and kissed him twice, once on each cheek with her soft lips. Makara was now officially in heaven! "The juice is fantastic, no?" she continued, sitting back down and smiling that award winning smile at Makara.

"Yeah, delicious!" he said, getting comfortable in his seat and enjoying the sunshine.

"Did you do the Dynamic Meditation?" she asked and took a mouthful of juice.

"Yeah, were you there too?" Makara questioned, wondering how on earth he could have missed her.

"Yes, I love that crazy Meditation," she continued,

in her cute accent and started laughing like a mad woman, taking Makara totally by surprise. After the shock passed, he joined her laughter and there they were, new friends, blissing out in the morning sun, drinking fresh juice.

It turned out that Citrine was from France and travelling Australia in her gap year. She was eighteen, didn't have a boyfriend and was an interesting, fun, good-looking young woman. Makara felt comfortable around her and the two of them really hit it off. He couldn't fully understand half the things she said but it didn't matter. He was in love and when she looked at him with those eyes and laughed, he was on another planet.

They ended up spending the whole day together. They chose the same workshops, swam in the river in the midday sun and even ended up having dinner. It was the longest first date ever! After dinner, Makara walked Citrine home to her tent and began getting very nervous. He'd had a few golden opportunities to kiss her during the day but for one reason or another hadn't taken them. He really, really wanted to kiss her.

"Goodnight Makara," Citrine said sweetly, standing at the entrance of her tent, planting a kiss on each of his cheeks. Makara moved in quickly for a hug and embraced her tightly, his sexual energy gathering force rapidly. Trying to remain somewhat calm, he breathed and relaxed a little, softening his grip on her.

He looked into Citrine's eyes and was now totally overtaken by his energy. Makara moved close to kiss her lips... they were soft and warm sending waves of pleasure through his body. He could feel his erection pressing against Citrine's leg and hoped she wouldn't notice. Once their tongues connected, Makara let his foot off the brake and dived in at a hundred miles per hour, his wild man taking over! He grabbed her tightly by the hips and started kissing her deeply with more strength. He had not kissed a woman for months and was so hungry, that he completely freaked Citrine out.

"Stop! Stop. Stop. Too much!" she cried loudly, pulling away from the embrace. Makara's whole energy shifted... instantly he felt awful.

"Sorry, I'm sorry..." he pleaded. Citrine angrily pressed him further away.

"What are you doing? It's too fast, you scare me," she said, backing away more, opening the zipper on her tent to get away. Makara was lost for words. He had gone from a wild tiger to a tiny mouse in seconds, and inside was not happy with himself at all.

"Listen. I'm sorry. I just couldn't help it," he stuttered, his guilt tearing him apart.

"Just go Makara... Please, just go."

He left not saying another word and walked home in the dark, totally off himself for ruining an epic day. He reflected on what had happened with Grace in the desert and how his energy just becomes so strong, that it's hard to control.

Maybe I'm not ready for all this self-pleasuring and raising my energy stuff, he questioned. Maybe I've got more than enough already?

18. A TASTE OF NIRVANA

Makara rolled over to turn off the alarm on his watch. It was still dark outside and instantly the memories of how much of an idiot he'd been the previous night came flooding back. He felt terrible. The Meditation was starting soon but he just lay there in bed, frozen, thinking that he was the worst person in the world. *What if Citrine's there this morning? What will I say?* he thought, feeling even more confused.

At the last minute, he realised he had a choice: to stay stuck in bed or snap out of it! Makara got up and ran to the Meditation Hall. For the next hour he breathed, screamed, stamped his feet and released so much anger and emotion, that by the end of it he came out a totally new man. He didn't even know if Citrine was there or not, 'cause the whole thing was done with a blindfold on.

During the process, Makara flashed on so many times in his life where he'd made himself wrong or belittled himself to try and not make others feel bad. This inner critic or this negative voice inside him had been uncovered and he made a decision then and there to never listen to this voice again. Its only purpose seemed to be to make him feel totally awful, so what was the point? If he was truly heading for a life of unlimited fun and joy, the sooner he brought awareness to those sorts of patterns, the better.

Back at the campsite, he slipped into the icy morning river for a swim to wash off the sweat from the Meditation. The sun was up a little way now and it was shaping up to be an excellent day. He joined Bob for breakfast outside the van and explained the whole situation from last night to him. Bob gave a new perspective on his sexual energy and explained what was right about it that he wasn't getting.

"This is your life force, your juice bro, and quite simply the more you have of it, the better your life's gunna be. And man, you've got a mountain of the stuff... look at you, you're so alive! All you need to do is master that energy and channel it wisely. The last thing you want to be doing is unexpectedly jumpin' on young women with it!" he said, laughing. "Men's sexual energy is like fire: it starts at the genitals and burns upwards, openin' the heart and the mind. As for women, it's the total opposite. Theirs is like water: it starts in the head and flows downwards through the heart and once their mind and heart are open, they will open sexually.

"It's just nuts, 'cause men fire up so quickly and it takes a while for the woman's water to heat up. More often than not, the man's volcano has erupted before the woman's water is even hot enough to make a cup of tea! It's about learnin' to be in that wild man energy and not having to race towards the finish line. You ought to come along with me to Tai Chi one mornin' man, that will help you a bunch!"

"Cheers mate. I feel I've a lot to learn and I really appreciate your wisdom and insights. Thanks."

Out of the blue, Citrine appeared. She looked even more beautiful than yesterday and Makara just about fell off his chair. There was a brief uncomfortable silence and then he sprang into action.

"Good morning Citrine! This is Bob, my really good friend."

Bob got up to meet her and knowing she was French, was ready for the double-kiss thing and also gave her a big-Bob-hair-everywhere-hug.

"Hello... I'm Citrine," she said quietly. Bob stood there admiring her beauty and looking into her sparkly eyes.

"What a beautiful young woman you are. Makara's told me lots of good things about you," he said, attempting to get his friend back in the good books. "I'll leave you guys to it. Time for me to go to Tai Chi," and he strolled off through the camping ground.

Citrine had Makara's jumper in her hand that he'd given her the previous night when she was cold.

"Here Makara. I wanted to give you this back," she said softly, still not quite looking him in the eyes.

"Look, I'm really sorry I jumped on you last night. I felt like a real idiot afterwards. It's been a long time since I've kissed a woman and I'm just so attracted to you, I couldn't help myself. I realise it shocked you. I'm sorry."

"Thank you for saying that," she said, now looking directly at him. "I am not used to this moving so quickly with a man, and I was not expecting it. You were like the jungle animal!" she continued in her broken English, letting out a sweet little giggle. "In France we do these things a wee bit different."

Makara was focused on her words and his heart had completely opened again. His confidence was rapidly returning and he looked at her with a cheeky grin: "Do you like jungle animals?" he questioned, trying to keep a straight face but laughing at the same time.

"Sometimes..." she replied, joining in the game. "It all depends on what animal it is."

The two of them hugged and laughed and it was all back on. He made her up a bowl of Bob's special muesli and some herbal tea, which she loved. They spent the morning at a creative acting and singing workshop that was absolutely fantastic. The grand finale was each person having to do a two minute solo performance in front of the group, which was challenging and fun at the same time. Makara did his very own Jim Morrison impersonation, which was explosive and left him shaking like a leaf afterwards.

Citrine and Makara spent another whole day together. They were both a little crazy in their own way and had a lot in common. They talked and talked, met people, played with a whole bunch of energised kids, danced and thoroughly squeezed the juice from the day. That night, when Makara walked Citrine home, they joked about the upcoming kiss and which animal he was going to be. It was such a relief for him that they could laugh about it. They hugged, shared a sweet little kiss and Makara went home to bed.

They had both been really getting a lot from the morning Meditation. All the emotional release was leaving Makara feeling much lighter, with a quiet mind. It was strange though, 'cause at the same time, he was feeling wobbly and vulnerable on a deeper level. Whatever was happening, it was a powerful process!

Citrine and Makara had made a plan to have breakfast together the following morning after Meditation. On the second day after Makara arrived at the festival, he had found a beautiful, secluded little spot up the river. The plan was to go there, have a swim and a sunrise breakfast.

Makara slept well and woke early before his alarm sounded. He was feeling bright-eyed and bushy-tailed. There was still half an hour before the Meditation, so he decided on some early morning self-pleasuring. He'd woken with an erection so it had pretty much automatically happened anyway. He was getting used to touching himself and had a small bottle of oil next to his bed which made the process a hundred times juicier. Slowly but surely he was enjoying his own body more and more. It was so liberating and the truth was, it was also love making practice, so when the time came, he would be prepared!

He saw Citrine on the way into the Meditation Hall and gave her a big hug. He was feeling so alive and so sexual; to just hold her was amazing. He could feel their warm bellies touching and her smell was different today. She smelt delicious and fruity. Once again through the Meditation, Makara moved internal mountains and was left with the same, blissful 'no mind' feeling. So relieving for the head to go on holidays for a while.

Back at camp he prepared a breakfast picnic with fruit, muesli, water and all the gear to eat it with. Citrine arrived with a blanket and a few other bits and pieces and away they went. They followed a track along the river bank, across a few beaches, under some huge, old trees and eventually came to the spot Makara had discovered earlier. It was like an untouched, private little slice of paradise. The river was gently running past and glistening, as the golden rays of the new day bounced off the water. They were pulled towards an area of green grass, lit up by the sun with some majestic big trees behind it.

Citrine lay out the blanket in a perfect spot and they decided on a swim. Makara was feeling free and as there was no one around, he stripped completely naked before running over and jumping in the river. Citrine casually removed all her clothes as well and wandered over to join him. Makara watched her enter the water, her whole body totally lit up in the morning sun. She was without a doubt the most beautiful woman he'd ever seen. The curves in her hips, her perfect breasts and the natural, easy way she carried herself was blowing Makara's mind... well, what was left of it! She also seemed so comfortable with being naked.

"Oohhh... it's freezing," giggled Citrine, as she entered the water. Makara began splashing her to the point where she was better off jumping in. She swam straight at him like an attack torpedo, grabbing his shoulders, laughing and trying to push him under. They wrestled and played for so long that they needed to get out, or freeze to death! Makara loved being naked with his new friend and enjoyed the short walk back to get the towels.

They dried off and put some warm clothes on. Before breakfast, Makara shared with Citrine what he'd learnt about gratitude and appreciation recently and they both chose five things each they were grateful for. He told her how he'd won the money and how the simple exercise of appreciation was changing his life. The breakfast was epic and the morning sun eventually began to warm them up. Citrine talked of her life in France, about her family and what she planned to study at university. It really didn't matter what she talked about, he just loved looking at her, listening to her and being around her sweet, fun vibration. The more they laughed together, the more his heart sang.

He was getting that strong feeling to kiss her again and this time, saw it coming early.

"My jungle animal is starting to wake up," he said, laughing at himself, while also honouring his energy at the same time. He decided on a new approach and lay down on his back on the blanket, surrendering to the energy. It was such a relief to let go and drop all expectations... of himself, of Citrine and whatever else his mind had planned out for him. The sun was much warmer now. So much so, he removed his T-shirt and just lay there soaking it up. He realised he didn't need to kiss Citrine, he didn't actually need to do anything. All he needed to do was enjoy what was happening right now. Enjoy his wild energy! How easy was that!

Sensing the ease in Makara and his total let go, Citrine moved close to him and began stroking his naked chest with her fingers. She was drawn to his fit, healthy body and the fact that he was no longer a threat, made room for her to express her sexual energy. She continued fondling his arms and running her fingers through his hair. Makara was smiling inside and out, receiving every bit of Citrine's loving touch. He felt his erection almost bursting out the top of his jeans but was totally relaxed about it. He'd been through that class already!

He squeezed his perineum, breathing the energy up out of his balls, put his tongue in place and let the energy flow down into his belly. Citrine was thoroughly enjoying herself and began to kiss his chest and shoulders. Makara was completely baffled and impressed at how well his technique of doing absolutely nothing was working. He began gently caressing her face and neck. It seemed as though her 'jungle animal' was waking up and he was loving every minute of it.

Their lips finally met and Citrine had never kissed him like she was kissing him now. She was now the one beginning to devour Makara and wanted his tongue... all of it! He grabbed the back of her pants and pulled her on top of him, their bodies immediately connecting. Makara continued running his hands across her back and sides. Citrine was kissing his face, his neck and even tongue-kissing his ear! He'd never been with a French woman before and it was really starting to get hot.

She was breathing heavily and starting to press her hips hard into Makara's sex. He could lie there no longer and flipped her over onto her back, letting his own jungle animal free. Citrine laughed and tried to wrestle him back down unsuccessfully. He pressed his body against hers and the kissing continued, getting hotter and hotter by the moment. Makara's body was now fully electrified with every cell buzzing at a million miles per hour.

The energy in his balls was getting intense and he breathed it up a few more times. He leaned back, lifting Citrine's shoulders off the blanket and ripped her shirt up over her head, exposing her lovely, full breasts, complete with two erect nipples. Makara stopped to admire them.

"Wow! You have such beautiful breasts," he said, and began kissing them and sucking on her nipples. Citrine breathed, moaned and laughed as Makara began kissing her all over. She reached down and opened the front of his jean's, exposing his throbbing, hot erection. This was the sign he was waiting for to totally set his 'wild man' free. He grabbed her by the hips and slid her pants off with ease.

Below him now, was the most ravishing vision he'd ever seen: a gorgeous, exploding, volcanic French woman, glowing with joy. Makara dragged his jeans off and took a deep breath, consciously slowing down a little and taking in the whole scene. Citrine pulled him back down onto her and continued kissing him like a wild woman. Their hot bodies were now dancing together, skin to skin. It was a phenomenal sight: two beautiful beings sharing their love and energy in the morning sunshine, next to a steadily flowing river. If heaven did exist on earth, then it was right here, right now.

Citrine was boiling over. "I want you inside me now!" she demanded, in a sweet but assertive way. Makara was taken by surprise, but he was prepared for this moment and reached over, pulling a condom from the pocket of his jeans. He took another big breath and just burst out laughing.

"And I was hesitant to let my jungle animal loose... you're on FIRE woman!" he said, fumbling around, making sure the condom was on properly.

Citrine was dripping wet and Makara slowly made small circles with the head of his penis around the outer lips of her vagina, entering her little by little. She moaned loudly and a bolt of lightning surged through Makara. They were now looking deep into each other's eyes and he gently moved his hips from side to side, in and out, slowly, respectfully moving deeper and deeper into Citrine. They continued kissing and caressing each other and time disappeared.

When the energy became too strong for Makara, he would draw it up his spine and back down into his belly. Citrine kept opening, drawing him in deeper and deeper, moaning and groaning as her pleasure reached new heights. It reached the point where he had so much energy moving through his body, that he didn't even feel like he had a body anymore. Suddenly, he felt like he'd completely disappeared. Their eyes met and they saw each other in a new light... it was as if neither of them were there, yet Makara felt so present at the same time.

His body began to tremble as the energy increased a hundred fold. Citrine began screaming orgasmically and her insides pulsed, sending rainbows of blissful lightning into Makara's burning erection and exploding heart. They'd become one, a trembling, orgasmic, pulsating, real-life sculpture of love making joy and freedom. Makara's whole body buckled rhythmically as he was entirely overtaken by something else and all he could do now was surrender to it. He took a deep breath, let go... and joined Citrine in her orgasmic cries.

19. COMING HOME

Dave opened his eyes and sat bolt upright in bed. Heart beating out of control and gasping for breath.

What the fuck? What's going on? Where the hell have I just been? His mind twisting in total disbelief, trying to get some sort of grip on the situation. His body was red hot and he could also feel a warm, sticky mess in his pyjama pants. He slowly lowered his body back down onto the bed and took a few full breaths.

Images of Citrine lying in the sun, flashed through his head. *Who is this woman?* Dave had three thousand questions and knew he had no answers. Normally this would frustrate him no end but something had changed. He felt okay with it and a little smile appeared on his face and he started to laugh.

He heard some noises coming from the kitchen

and figured his parents must've been awake. Dave reached up, pulling open his curtains and had the second big shock of the morning. Beyond the fences and the back neighbour's house, was a huge rainbow. Some light rain was falling and the morning sun had created a colourful arch of joy. Dave flashed on his dream, recalling the rainbows and felt a sense of peace wash over him.

He lay there, breathing, admiring the rainbow and piece by piece recollecting the journey he'd just been on. He felt like he'd been asleep for a whole year; so much had happened yet it was only one night. Memories started flooding in. Dave reached over and grabbed a pen and paper from his desk. He began madly scribbling down words and phrases. By the time he'd written one down, another was at the front of his mind. *Listen to my body. Rest when I'm tired. Stop eating crap. Go surfing now. Hang out with Bob more. Go travelling. Quit my job. Life's about having fun. Get over the whole serious thing.* He couldn't believe how all this stuff was just coming through him but every time he wrote something down, it rang true and goose bumps tingled all over his body.

Gratitude. Appreciation. Celebrate my sexual energy. Pleasure myself. Dance without drinking. Spend time with amazing, open people. Travel, travel, travel. Let loose my creativity. My entrepreneur. Dave just kept on writing. The more he wrote, the better he began to feel. The energy that was moving through his body was new and refreshing. The old, sick, tired Dave that had gone to sleep the previous night had 'left the building'. Who knows where he'd gone and it didn't really matter, but the young man who'd taken his place was very much alive, empowered and ready to grab his life by the balls!

Outside his room, the rainbow had now faded and a gentle, Sunday morning sun shower was taking place. Dave filled two pages before he knew it, of inspirational tips and ways to make his life better. He reflected on the dramas of the past few months and could see so clearly where he'd been stuck. Holding onto his ex-girlfriend, hating his job at the hardware, trying to fit in with all his old friends and totally consumed with his mystery sickness. He was also now aware of the steps he needed to take to reclaim his life.

Dave felt strong and clear. It was as if he'd gone from one extreme to the next overnight. He was feeling incredible, so grateful for his new insights and seeing things differently. It was bizarre; he could see the positive sides of everything he thought about. Something had shifted deeply within him and he felt the need to anchor this whole new perception of the world as best he could. He grabbed a new sheet of paper and decided to write himself a letter, just in case he was still dreaming or this new awareness was temporary. Either way, he needed something to remind him and he had to do it now.

Dear Dave,
Whatever just happened to you last night seems to have changed your life forever. Please remember

always that you are an amazing man, full of energy, gifts and creativity to share with the world. It is time for you to stand up and become all that you were put on this earth to be. It is time to appreciate and be grateful for yourself and everything in your life. Let go of the serious, hard ways and embrace the joy, the freedom, the love and the dance that this life really is. And trust it. What if your whole purpose here was to enjoy yourself? You have even been given a new name, MAKARA. Use this now as a reminder of your joy and when the time comes you can fully embrace it as your new name.

Dave was holding the pen, shaking, looking for more words to finish his letter when he heard the scream of a familiar bird outside and immediately looked up. A huge, black cockatoo was passing over the house and heading in the direction of where the rainbow had just been. Its ancient cries echoed through Dave's body as he watched it disappear into the distance.

"This is all way too weird!" he declared to himself out loud and decided to get out of bed. He didn't even know what was real anymore, his dream had been so vivid... and then the rainbow... the cockatoo... the boundaries between realities were fading fast.

He'd started on some new medication a few days back and thought that could be to blame. They all had different side effects but none had ever been as uplifting, real and expanding as this. It was hard to say what it was. Possibly he was just losing his mind? As

Dave went to stand up he noticed a sparkly, light-brown coloured stone on the carpet next to his bed. It was about the size of a twenty cent piece and an uneven shape. He picked it up to examine it more closely, fully puzzled and positive it wasn't there when he'd gone to bed the previous night! *Can this day get any weirder?* he thought, tentatively removing his pyjama pants and trying to not get fresh sperm all over his legs.

A shower was always good to get some early morning clarity. He walked down the hallway and flashed on the number of Sunday mornings he'd stumbled into the bathroom to vomit the contents of a poisoned party stomach from the previous night. Right now, those days seemed long gone and he had a feeling that he would never suffer from a hangover again. The shower helped a bit and one thing became clear: he needed to see Bob as soon as possible.

As he turned to leave the bathroom he caught a glimpse of himself in the mirror. It shocked him and he stopped, leaning in to get a full, 'up close' view of himself. To be very honest, he hardly even recognised the young man he was staring at. His eyes had definitely changed and the skin on his face even looked different... it was the colour or something. Dave stood still, looking into his own eyes and liked what he was looking at. A smile blossomed on his face and he had an unmistakeable feeling that everything was going to be okay. He'd never looked at himself like that before, ever.

Dave had breakfast with his parents, which was

also very strange. He felt so different and it was as though he hadn't seen them in a long time. They even looked different as well and both mentioned a couple of times how well Dave looked. There was absolutely no tension in the air. It was the classic, relaxed Sunday morning family breakfast.

His mum and dad weren't on his case and everyone just seemed happy doing their own thing. Dave observed what was happening and felt extremely content. Another insight from the dream catapulted into his mind. *The world is a reflection of you*, he thought to himself and this was exactly what was taking place in front of him. *Is this really how it works?* he questioned, feeling surprised and shovelling in the last spoonful of breakfast.

The morning was slipping away and the movie store would be opening shortly. Bob always worked the Sunday morning shift and Dave had so much to share with him, he couldn't wait to get there. He gathered up his morning notes, the video to return, plus the stone he'd found next to his bed, brushed his teeth and was out the door.

The rain had eased and the clouds were breaking up to reveal a sunny day. Dave felt comfortable in his little car and was also very happy he didn't have to work today. As far as the hardware went, he also knew deep down his days there were numbered. With his new-found awareness, he figured simply that anything that wasn't bringing him joy, he would be letting go of.

As predicted, Bob's Kombi was parked outside

the store and it warmed Dave's heart to see it. Again he flashed on his dream and all the adventure's they'd had in that wild, old van.

"Aloha Dave," Bob said, sounding super chirpy as he walked in the door. Dave stood there for a while with a huge smile on his face, deeply happy to see Bob again. He looked for ages until he realised he was probably weirding him out and figured he'd better say something.

"Mornin' Bob," he replied enthusiastically. The store was completely empty and naturally as anything, he walked towards Bob with open arms, ready for a hug. Bob responded warmly and the two of them embraced like brothers.

"Hey, you feelin' better today man?" Bob asked, still concerned about his young friend.

"Yeah... much better, thanks mate. I feel like a new man today."

Bob smiled at Dave, nodding his head with knowing eyes.

"Awesome man... So how was Tarzan?"

"It was a beauty, thanks. It actually left me feelin' great and had some quality messages about life," Dave replied.

"Speakin' of messages about life!" Bob announced. "I've had a few amazin' ones in the last few days myself and have actually made some big decisions. Apparently there's been somethin' big goin' on astrologically, a really powerful time... I've realised I'm wastin' my life away in this damn movie store so I'm finishin' up in two weeks and I'm going back to California.

My brother's got this boomin' business goin' on and a property he needs help with, and I haven't seen my family for years. It's feelin' like a time on the planet where you need to follow your intuition, your dreams and your joy, so that's what I'm gunna do bro!"

Dave was staring at him blankly. *Quitting his job? Going on an adventure?? Spending time helping his brother out???*

"You alright dude?" Bob enquired, a little concerned about his young mate. "It looks like you've seen a ghost or somethin'... you're not gunna pass out on me again are ya?"

"Nah, all good mate. My health feels solid this mornin'... I'm just havin' a really strange day, that's all. I had this dream last night..." Dave paused and felt sharing his dream right now would just make things weirder and weirder, so he decided to stop. Putting his hand into his pocket, he pulled out the stone he'd found earlier.

"Any idea what this is?" he questioned, changing the subject and handing the small, sparkly rock over to Bob.

"Yeah bro, that's a piece of Citrine." Dave's heart exploded and a rush of energy passed through his body, his mind now in total malfunction. *That was her name, that was her name!* he thought to himself excitedly. Bob went on, not taking so much notice of Dave's strange behaviour anymore: "It's a precious stone or crystal or whatever you want to call it, but one of its key properties is that it can't hold any negative energy," he said, handing it back to Dave. "Give it a go. See if you can think of something negative."

Dave stood there, completely still, in shock, holding onto the little honey-coloured pebble. *How on earth did this end up in my room?* He began to question his sanity again and quickly realised that wasn't the best direction to go in. Bob sensed Dave was struggling, the look on his face a dead give away that his mind was spinning out of control. He moved closer to Dave and put his hands on his shoulders to try and help ground him back into his body.

"You know Dave, sometimes when life gets really complicated and weird and we try to make sense of it, it actually makes it worse. Take a deep breath in... slowly breathe out... feel your feet on the ground and just surrender to the mystery of it all. Especially now, things seem to be getting so intense on planet earth and the more we can say goodbye to our minds and hello to our hearts, the better off we're all gunna be."

Bob's words hit the spot and Dave's mind started to let go... he could even feel his body beginning to relax. It was like magic and he instantly felt much better.

"Thanks mate, my mind just goes bananas sometimes. I liked that bit about surrenderin' to the mystery too. Reckon that's a real key for my life." He sat down on a little stool beside the counter and looked up at Bob with a peaceful smile.

Bob laughed and said passionately:

"And I've got some other good news for ya! My blue bus is gunna be up for sale and I'm lookin' for her to go to a good home... Would you be interested in an upgrade?" A cheeky smile came across his face and he began to laugh again. He looked Dave straight in the eyes, "She really is a ticket to freedom ya know!"

Thank You for taking the time
to read my first book.
You will be very happy to know that:

10% of all book profits go to
The Margaret River Surfrider Foundation

They are a local community branch of Surfrider Australia, that are dedicated to protecting the waves and beaches of this precious coastal region which I call home.

To order more copies of this fantastic book go to:
www.vividpublishing.com.au/makara

For more information about Douglas Cooney, future books and the transformational, 'A taste of freedom' weekend retreats, visit his Facebook Author page.

The money used to publish this book was 'Crowd funded' through www.pozible.com

A HUGE Thank you to everyone that pledged towards my campaign and helped to make it happen. The support and encouragement I received was overwhelming and I am super grateful.

I would also like to acknowledge and thank my amazing parents. Mum for her care, patience and huge help in proof reading this book. Dad for his financial support, strength and providing an adventurous childhood. I am eternally grateful and love you both very much!

MAJOR CONTRIBUTORS

Ralph & Amanda Cooney	Rosa Ralli
Angela Macqueen	Micheal O'Keefe
Elise Savaresse	Dan Marsden
Anthony Bell	The Howard Family
Elisabeth Jackson	Sam Macqueen
Anna & Brad Marriott	Paula Amorim
Ben & Aimee Cooney	Chris Tague
Peter & Sally Davies	Severine Maudoux
Prem Gitika	Nathan Psaila
Lotti St.Clair	Aaron Lumsdaine
David Webster	Shane Moody

THANK YOU

Pamela Forward
Flynn & Dylan Cooney
Jake Graebner-Bond
Matthew Learmonth
David Chick
Chontelle Balbi
Matthew Smith
Summer and Anne (Team Taiwan)
Greg Wilson
Kristy Joy Brown